The
Making of
Tomorrow's
Physician:

Heart of the Art — My Way

A Unique Approach to
Medical Student Teaching

Joel S. Zaretzky M.D.

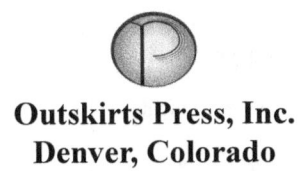

Outskirts Press, Inc.
Denver, Colorado

This book is dedicated to all the students I've taught and mentored: May they be my legacy. I also dedicate this book to my loving wife, Patricia, whose patience and support have helped me practice the wonderful art of teaching medicine.

The Making of Tomorrow's Physician: Heart of the Art — My Way
A Unique Approach to Medical Student Teaching
All Rights Reserved.
Copyright © 2009 Joel S. Zaretzky M.D.
Edited by Sharlene L. Kehlenbeck
v3.0

Outskirts Press, Inc.
http://www.outskirtspress.com

ISBN: 978-1-4327-3489-3

Library of Congress Control Number: 2009929584

Outskirts Press and the "OP" logo are trademarks belonging to Outskirts Press, Inc.

PRINTED IN THE UNITED STATES OF AMERICA

Contents

The Making of Tomorrow's Physician:
The Heart of the Art—My Way!

By Joel S. Zaretzky, M.D., P.C.

Dr. Zaretzky is an Assistant Professor of Medicine, Yale University School of Medicine, New Haven, Connecticut. He is also Chairman of the Ambulatory Care Residency Program Curriculum Design Committee for Griffin Hospital, Derby, Connecticut. In 1999, Dr. Zaretzky received the Ambulatory Professor of the Year Award for Medical Student Teaching from Yale University.

The practice of medicine is an art that is based in science. What has been lost in clinical medical student teaching is the humanism that puts the "heart" into the job. Just as it is vital that the doctor see the patient as a whole person, not simply as a problem to solve, it is equally important that the teaching physician view the medical student as an individual, and strive to nurture that student's best qualities. This I call finding the student's seeds of growth.

Over the past 30 years, I have taught over a thousand medical student ambulatory care clinical rotations and through this experience have developed my four-week teaching model. This book presents the basics needed to develop the fledgling M.D. into a mature "student doctor." I hope this book, and the methods within it, inspire both students and physicians to learn something new and to reach the doctor's ultimate goal: to better his fellow man.

CHAPTER **1**

First Sight

The song "Getting to Know You" is a very appropriate way to begin this chapter. It is extremely important for the doctor or attending (that is, the teaching physician) to take the time to get to know the medical students as he guides them through the next four weeks. I like to go over their backgrounds, interests, and schools attended, and as we size each other up I can start to determine what qualities I see in each student that I can utilize in his or her growth. Every student is different, and their backgrounds are quite diversified— they may have been English, history, or music majors instead of the more commonly seen science majors. Many of the students I've spent time with have worked for a number of years after college, bringing with them a special kind of maturity. I take this information into consideration as we begin our time together.

In turn, I also think it's important for the attending to share a bit about his or her daily life outside the office. Does he have to pick up his children at school at the end of the day? How does she actually juggle a career with the other parts of her day-to-day life? How does he handle the additional stressors in his day, such as insurance company issues and all the important telephone calls that have to be made? Of course, the teaching physician doesn't have to share all the specifics of his life, but opening up a little helps the students see him as a whole person, someone who has many other things to do in addition to taking care of sick patients.

The Big Question

One of the first questions I ask my medical students is: "Why did you want to become a physician?" The student's answer can be very revealing. I have received answers ranging from "My grandmother wanted me to" or "I like biology" to "I want to be a surgeon because I like using my hands." Some even mention financial motives. The best answer, in my opinion, is "I want to better my fellow man." I teach my students that the most important thing they can do each day is to look in the mirror and ask: "What am I going to do today?" and to answer: "I am going to help someone who is less fortunate." There is nothing more satisfying than helping someone with a problem, whether that problem is as simple as mild anxiety or a skin lesion, or as complicated and difficult as cancer. Recently, a medical student from Kenya illustrated this truth to me when he mentioned that he had cared for his very ill mother in Africa for many years. This experience led him to the knowledge that he wanted to be a physician and make a difference in society.

I have heard that many doctors are actually discouraging their children from entering the medical profession, due to the long hours, high responsibilities, medical legal aspects, and insurance issues. It is true that these are all part of being a doctor, but as I say to my medical students, this is also true: You will make a difference in your patients' lives. Something you might say or do during your day could change the course of someone's life. You are in charge of their medical and possibly psychological care. This is a special gift. Understanding this truth may actually give direction to the student doctor and underscore why she decided to enter medical school. If she can grasp this concept and begin to transform into an individual who can heal by her very presence, I have done my job. Nothing can stop her now, not even the daily pressures of the modern ambulatory care setting. If she can help someone else, she can better the world.

CHAPTER 2

The First Two Weeks

Initial Discussion

The first meeting with the student is really an overview of what he can expect during the rotation. After he meets the staff (an important part of the first day, since the success of the rotation will depend in part on how well the student interacts with other staff members) and takes a tour of the office to help him become oriented, we sit down to go over the syllabus. I have constructed a detailed syllabus (see an example in *Figure 1*) that outlines a typical four-week primary care rotation in my office. During the initial discussion, we go over this information, including the specific schedule of the rotation and how much time will be spent at the medical school for didactic sessions as well as at the clinic. We discuss what is expected in the physician's notes, so the student begins to understand how detailed and extensive notes have to be in the complex medical insurance society of the 21st century. The syllabus also includes a guide for each type of office visit, such as urgent care, revisits, and complete physicals, as well as house calls and hospital visits. We go over what will be expected from the student regarding day-to-day requirements in patient care. The student is told that there will be a weekly three-hour conference during which specially prepared clinical cases will be discussed and tests will be given, and that he will have all the information needed to perform these tests several days prior to the discussion. The tests will parallel the learning of the student in the rotation, and are selected to better him as the total physician. Each student will be required to take several cases as a student doctor, in which he will make decisions that will affect his patients' lives and the quality of their health. We talk about the weekly and biweekly critiques of the student that will take place, and discuss the qualities they will be evaluated on. The students are notified that they will be required to maintain the pace of the busy medical office and should take appropriate time in the rooms, but I am also sure to mention that it takes many years of practice to perfect this art. At this time, I also ask the student if there are any specific topics he'd like to see addressed during the rotation, so I can tailor the program to fit his needs. I believe having a written recommended program gives the rotation a structure that the student truly requires at this stage of his development. With a busy waiting room, multiple phone calls, and important diagnoses and treatments being discussed, the syllabus helps to structure the student's day.

Attached to the syllabus is a list of important medical topics to be used as a general course of reading. On a daily basis, the student needs to do background reading on each of his cases, but his independent learning is supplemented with additional articles. I give each student 8 or 10 articles per week that truly reinforce the required learning on the cases he has seen during the week. The students are encouraged to keep these articles as part of their personal library. Although each student receives articles dealing with front-line primary care topics such as sinusitis, headaches, chest pain, pneumonia, asthma, hypertension, diabetes mellitus, chronic lung disease, and colon cancer, I also keep in mind the specific interests of the student. If a urology resident is part of the rotation, for example, I might select articles dealing with bladder cancer, renal cancer, cystitis, urethritis, or prostate problems. (While I'm gathering these articles, I also might be learning something new—as physicians, we can learn from our students!)

The previous rotations of each student are diverse. Some have only done psychiatry; some have had more experience, such as an internal medicine rotation, surgery rotation, or even other primary care rotations. Clearly, those with prior rotation experience will find it easier to be successful with this rotation. However, I have found that even those who have only had a psychiatry rotation (of course, an extremely important part of the total care of each patient) still do extremely well in this multifaceted program. Of major importance in my initial discussion with the students who will be with me for the next four weeks is to stress that my ultimate goal is to make this student the best doctor he or she can be. In order to do so, I will be a coach on the sidelines. I strive to instill excitement in the student, and the only way to do so is to show how excited I am about teaching a student of his or her caliber. May the teaching begin!

The Student Enters the Examining Room

The first two weeks of the rotation are truly a growth phase. The student gains the confidence to enter the examining room, introduce himself ("Good morning. My name is Mr. Smith and I am a medical student at Yale working with Dr. Z."), and truly take charge of the office visit. If the student is to do so, it is vital that he is not thought of as a "shadow," but rather as a student doctor. The "shadow" does not learn much, in my view. He is just watching another individual do his work. He cannot grow as a student to become a student doctor and, eventually, a competent physician.

The student is told upon arrival that he is in charge of each patient to whom he was assigned. Whether that patient is an urgent office visit, a house call, or is in a nursing home, the student is responsible for any and all workups, including laboratory data, CAT scans, X-rays, and preventive screening methods. Thus, the student doctor will perform the initial physical exam on a new patient and will order the laboratory and preventive screening tests. (He is, of course, taught that another female member of the staff must always be present during a breast or gynecological exam of a female patient, and that this should be marked in the progress note.) The student doctor will be the medical authority to his patients. After each patient is seen, he will come out of the room and present the case to me in as much detail as possible (in an enclosed area due to HIPPA laws). Although, as a mentor, I am right by the student's side with every decision and every lab data ordered, it is important that he begins to see himself as the health-care worker in charge. This helps him develop his individual style and confidence. As the teaching physician, I remain for the most part a silent observer, watching the student's physical examination technique, noting the patient's reaction to what the student says during the visit, and evaluating the student's directive questioning skills.

Time constraints are always a concern. The waiting room might be very busy, with people waiting perhaps an hour or more as the student attempts to direct the patient to obtain the appropriate information with which to construct a differential diagnostic plan. The syllabus is a helpful tool to aid the student in understanding what a brief, intermediate, or extended visit and complete physical entails; however, any excess time in the room is never counted against the medical student. It takes time to learn the appropriate way of directing the patient to reveal the necessary information. He must learn the importance of listening, then intervening when necessary to redirect the patient. Performing a problem-oriented, focused exam, without taking over the history and not letting the patient speak, is a learned skill. He is beginning to learn how to establish a rapport with the patient, as well as gaining the confidence needed to take an adequate history or perform a physical exam. In the beginning, students are often overwhelmed by the realization that taking proper notes that abide by the "laws of insurance" is as important as taking the patient's history and the exam itself. By the second week of the rotation, however, the student can usually adapt, although he may need to stay a little later in the day to finish up these notes. Finally, the student learns that every day brings a unique set of problems. If you take into consideration the family dynamics of each patient, and the difficulties inherent in living in the 21st century, the office setting can seem more complicated than a soap opera, with each visit bringing a new set of characters.

At the end of each day it is important to sit down with each student and ask, "How was your day? What are the problems you are having going into the room? Is there anything I can do to make it easier for you?" My task as a mentor is to make that student the best physician he or she can be. It is vital that the student understand that during the four-week rotation he is not a person looking in from the outside, but rather he is the reason why I am there. We are taking care of the patient as a team. Once the student realizes the importance of his role, he becomes a huge asset to the health-care team, not an extra task for the primary doctor.

Arriving on "The Set"

A term I often use throughout the rotation is "the student actor." What do I mean by that? In the beginning, the student must take on the role of physician. When she enters the office at the start of the rotation, she is actually arriving on "the set." She needs to present herself as a complete physician, with the professionalism, sensitivity to the feelings of others, and intellectual capabilities necessary to carry out the difficult task of caring for the patient and all of his complicated problems. There will come a day when the student truly is that physician, but first she must be an actor in that role. It is helpful to the student actor, at least at first, to be somewhat mechanistic. In other words, she should have an agenda, or an outline of the patient visit, before she enters the examining room. That outline will help direct the visit for maximum efficiency. The patient will begin to think of her as "the doctor" when she looks the part; her professionalism is developing as well as her competence, and she requires less total supervision. It is not uncommon for patients who have been followed by my fine rotating medical students to call and ask specifically for "Jack" or "Wendy." This is because these students have begun making the transformation from student actor to physician. To the patient, they have become a trusted individual whom the patient can rely on for the potential resolution of his medical, social, and psychological issues. But before the student can be a true teacher to her patients, she must be believable in the acting role. I often tell my students: Believe in yourself and others will believe in you.

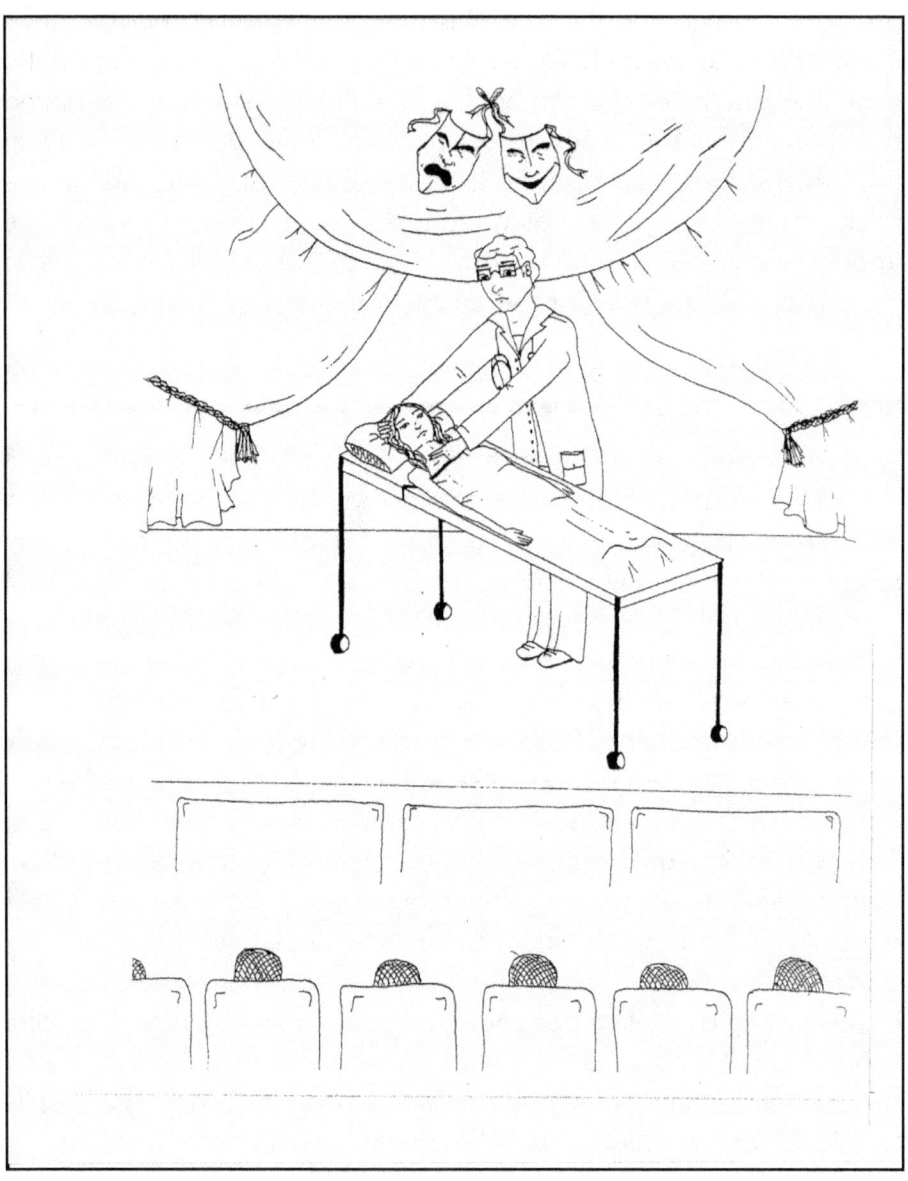

The student actor takes the stage.

Individual Technique

My goal as I stand to the side in the examining room and watch the student as he takes the patient's history is not necessarily for him to duplicate my style as a doctor. I want these student doctors to develop their own special technique with their patients. My technique is to be somewhat familiar with each patient, to know their families, their hobbies, even upcoming family engagements. I find this to be quite helpful in enabling the patient to tell me everything that's on her mind; with this approach, even deep-seated private issues seem easier for the patient to divulge. But it is important that each student develop his own technique, and I allow this to happen. I am very pleased when I see the student "come into himself" as a doctor, and not conform to anyone else's style.

CHAPTER 3

The Busy Ambulatory Setting

For many years, I have watched medical students arriving at my office for the first time; it is similar to watching someone parachuting into the jungle—it's a whole different world! Obviously, every ambulatory office setting is different. The medical student may land in settings as diverse as hospital clinics, primary office settings in family practice and internal medicine, pediatric offices, surgical, or OB/GYN. Each office has its own character and flow, and each has its own inherent problems and different personalities. The primary doctor himself is working under a pressure that far exceeds that of taking care of patients. Each office, of course, has a waiting room, front desk, business office, and examining rooms, and each in turn has its own unique personality that the medical student needs to adjust to. There may be other doctors, other medical students, nurses, nurse practitioners, PAs, medical assistants, and vital office administrative staff. In spite of all these important people, it is imperative that the student is taught that he or she is of the utmost importance and is seen at all times as a vital member of the health-care team and not, as previously mentioned, a "shadow."

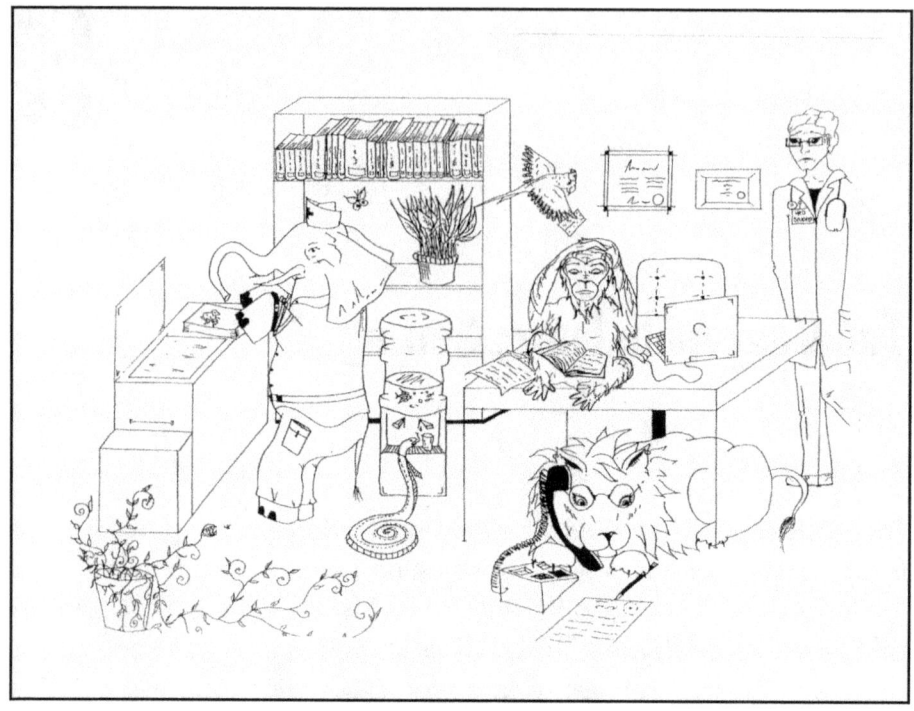

Welcome to the jungle!

Phone Calls

The intervals in the ambulatory setting are filled with telephone calls; filling out forms such as physical exams, appointment schedules, school physicals, and other reports; and inquiries. These duties of the physician may go on after hours and it is likely that they will often have to be taken home for completion. This is an excellent teaching modality for students. I encourage them to not only call the patient the day after the visit to see how they are doing, but also to take an active role in that patient's total care. Prior to the phone call, the student has reviewed any tests that have been performed, such as X-rays or echocardiograms, and has considered his initial impressions and any research he did after seeing the patient. He has made his interpretations based on these impressions and on the results of the tests, has presented his findings to me, and we have discussed diagnosis and treatment plans in detail. The student will call the patient to go over this information, and possibly to schedule a follow-up visit. If the patient has had an abnormal chest X-ray, for example, a larger-scale plan is necessary, and a follow-up visit is required. Thus, the student doctor is truly taking over the case. He is feeling an independence that most students don't seem to find in their other rotations. He begins to gain confidence and competence by making decisions, right or wrong, regarding the patient's care (of course, I am there to help guide the student to the right decision if necessary). This encounter by telephone is a win–win situation for both the student doctor and the patient.

Additional Duties

It is important that students feel useful throughout the day, that they are true members of the team, even if they are not at that moment working with patients in the "student doctor" capacity. There are many other service-specific procedures that students can perform in the office. In addition to retrieving charts and bringing patients to the examining room, they can answer the phone and take appointments. Supervised students can administer vitamin B12 and testosterone injections, and once trained by a technician, can perform EKGs. With supervision, they can help register patients. The staff usually retrieves lab results, but the student can assist here as well. Lastly, a meeting with the business manager to discuss various business aspects and diagnostic coding can be highly valuable.

CHAPTER 4

Finding the Beauty in Each Patient

One of the most important lessons I can impart to my students is for them to discover the beauty within each of their patients. I teach my students that no matter what the person's outside appearance, each one possesses a special, unique beauty waiting to be discovered. This has nothing to do with their clothing or personal hygiene, but with their value as a person. The physician must look at each patient with respect, and concentrate on their humanistic qualities in order to realize that they are dealing not only with diagnoses on paper, but with a total human being. As such, they need to get rid of their own biases, obviously racial biases or those against sexual orientation, but also against people who may be drug addicts or possibly even drug dealers. When a doctor sits in judgment of a patient, it impairs his ability to heal him.

The Total Patient

As part of looking at the patient as a whole, students are taught to familiarize themselves with the patient's family unit. Perhaps someone's sister is in some type of trouble or a mother is very ill with cancer—it's important for the student to understand the effects of these situations on the patient. They are taught the importance of reviewing socioeconomic issues, and looking into any psychological issues or troublesome family dynamics in order to provide complete treatment. I tell my students to try to think like Sherlock Holmes in this regard: Investigate every possibility to "solve" the case. For instance, a patient may be suffering from fatigue and insomnia due to anxiety. By determining the source of the anxiety, such as situational issues of domestic violence or mental abuse, the student has the information necessary to direct the patient to get help. The students are diagnosticians of any problems a complex individual might have, whether it's psychiatric issues, such as depression, or trying to discern reasons for weight loss, such as cancer. Their self esteem is enhanced as they realize the power they possess to help someone. They are performing an extremely important service to humanity by taking care of their fellow man. My role as mentor is to help them become excited about their vital work in the practice of medicine. With this outlook, any subject they study will be exciting.

One of the "pearls of wisdom" in patient care that I like to instill in my students involves this concept of seeing the patient not just as a name or a number, but rather as a total person. I tell my students to try to find something unique about each patient and write this specific detail in his or her chart. Mrs. Smith, for example, may have a special interest, such as knitting or going on trips. She may have a sister named Betty or may even have spent time in a concentration camp long ago. Taking the time to find out some detailed, not general, information helps the physician see the patient as an individual. On the next office visit, when she asks how the patient's cough is, she can also inquire about her sister Betty or her trip to Hawaii. If, in the course of the conversation, the patient mentioned an important event going on in her life, such as a wedding, bar mitzvah, or 25th wedding anniversary, the doctor can ask how it went. When the student doctor, and eventually physician, takes the time to familiarize herself with the patient, she is seen as a person and not as someone standing on a pedestal.

One student of mine, Sarah, was charmed by a 75-year-old Scottish patient. As Sarah took her patient's history, she took the time to find out something personal about her, learning a bit of the patient's cultural background in the process. In a charming Scottish accent, the patient told Sarah about Scotland's New Year's tradition, "Who first foot the house?" It seems that if a tall, dark-haired member of the family rings the bell and takes the first step into the house at midnight, good luck will follow. He traditionally brings with him a loaf of bread, silver for wealth, a drink, and money in his pocket. What a fascinating tradition! Sarah was happy to learn about it, and by doing so, was able to develop a wonderful rapport with her patient, establishing the important sense of trust. This patient had actually been fearful of doctors in the past because she was afraid of what they might find. But because of Sarah's encouragement, she went through with her lab work and further testing. The patient had come to the office because of extreme fatigue; Sarah's "Sherlock Holmes" thinking helped her diagnose the patient with severe vitamin B12 deficiency and Hashimoto's disease. She also educated this patient on what she would need to do to be healthy in the future, including serial lab work such as cholesterol, urine testing, and electrocardiogram. The patient did go on to have the recommended colonoscopy, mammogram, bone densitometry, and other tests. Sarah's rotation ended the next day, but she asked to be notified of the results of the tests she had ordered. Her patient ended up having colon cancer, which was treated with resection. Sarah had saved a life. She'll carry that honor for the rest of her life. The student doctor had truly arrived when she asked for those results. Who first foot the house? In this case, Sarah took the first step toward becoming a true healer. Who knows? Maybe she had a little Scottish in her. Maybe she found the beauty of medicine.

CHAPTER **5**

Essential Qualities

Compassion ▬▬▬▬▬▬▬▬▬▬▬▬▬▬▬▬▬▬▬▬▬▬▬▬

In addition to medical expertise, I also look for the development of some perhaps less definable, but no less important, characteristics in my students. The first of these is compassion. One of my students, Jennifer H., exemplified this quality. It was 4 p.m. on the last day of Jennifer's rotation, and the staff were exchanging goodbyes with this very fine student. It came to Jennifer's attention that a patient she had seen previously, an elderly man named Jay, was sitting in the waiting room because he wanted to ask her a question. Although Jay could have been seen by someone else, Jennifer took the time in this last patient encounter of her rotation to go out into the waiting room and bring this gentleman in to an examining room. She truly displayed the compassion and conscientiousness that I like to see in a student at this stage of the rotation. Obviously, the doctor–patient rapport was there because Jay absolutely felt that Jennifer was his doctor. Jennifer had seen him for several visits through her rotation for benign prostatic hyperplasia (BPH), depression, an upper respiratory infection, and dizziness, as well as speaking with him multiple times on the phone. Jay's depression stemmed from the loss of his wife 20 years previously: They had been in the coronary care unit at the same time for myocardial infarction; he was sent for a coronary artery bypass and survived, but his wife didn't make it. Jennifer had displayed compassion in caring for the well being of this patient, and on that afternoon, continued to do so. She initially thought it was a possibility Jay was seeking help because of anxiety or depression, but when she brought him into the examining room, he complained of dizziness and stated that he had a spinning sensation. There was no chest pain or palpitations. After performing an exam, she informed me that his blood pressure was slightly low and he was dizzy, and that she had decided to do an EKG. I entered the examining room while it was being performed and realized that Jay's heart rate was 30. Showing tremendous kindness, Jennifer volunteered to drive the patient to the hospital herself. Of course, we decided that it was best to call for an ambulance to take him to the hospital, where he had a permanent pacemaker inserted by his cardiologist. Jennifer's sixth sense, caring, and compassion saved Jay's life. A medical student with character had made a difference.

When I think of students with compassion, I also remember Jim, a 44-year-old man who decided later in life to specialize in psychiatry after spending 14 years as a psychiatric technician and administrator at a major institution. Jim would spend many hours with his patients, even taking up to 45 minutes for an intermediate visit. He had an ability to comfort each patient in a special way; in particular I remember his compassion with a patient suffering from ALS, and his support for that patient's family. Jim was amazed by the number of patients in the primary care setting who had a need for some sort of psychiatric care; he found it very surprising that up to 60% of patients displayed psychiatric issues, and that these issues were left to the primary care physician rather than a psychiatrist. In conjunction with Jim's highly developed sense of compassion, his meticulous methods of examination also uncovered a good amount of pathology. For instance, after performing a complete physical on a patient of mine, he came out to tell me that there was a suspicious lesion on the patient's upper back, and subsequently performed a biopsy with me in the office. This lesion proved to be a malignant melanoma, which was later fully excised by a surgeon. Finding this cancer gave Jim a tremendous sense of satisfaction. I give him full credit for saving this patient's life. The care and compassion that he displayed for his patients during his rotation with me, including their family issues and social and psychological needs, continue for this student, who is now in psychiatric residency. He had a taste of the requirements needed to be a fine total physician in the 21st century. He learned this in the all-important ambulatory care setting. Clearly, he was on the front line of medicine.

Empathy

I encourage my students to look into their own histories, both personal and medical, so they can uncover areas that will help them in understanding their patients. This quality, of course, is called empathy. When a doctor is empathetic toward his patient, the patient will always benefit—it becomes much easier for the doctor to develop a good rapport with the patient and his family. The quality of empathy gives the student doctor more of a "database" to work with so he can help solve the problems of his patients.

I'd like to use the experience of Bill, a 28-year-old medical student, to illustrate the importance of this quality. Bill's cousin had been murdered in New York City during an armed robbery a few years previously. The patient he was seeing had just lost his 24-year-old son due to a drug overdose. Bill utilized his concern and empathy for this gentleman by remembering from his own experience that the patient's suffering was an ongoing process. He was able to offer the patient help from many different avenues, including antidepressant medication and supportive psychotherapy, in addition to being a source of comfort and kindness. Bill learned how important it is to use his heart as well as his medical knowledge. This patient had been lost, and with Bill's help was able to begin working through his grief. Bill began to understand an important element of the art of healing.

Another student of mine who had been diagnosed with cancer

of the GU tract and had been forced to take a year off from school for chemotherapy showed tremendous empathy toward patients in the office who had similar problems. This student displayed true compassion, a beautiful rapport, and tremendous empathy toward these patients and their families. They say that when a physician has been a patient himself, he is able to handle his patients in a perhaps more sympathetic way. Maybe he is able to truly treat them as he would like to be treated. The proverb "Do unto others as you would have them do unto you" has special meaning to the physician.

Vigilance

Vigilance is a necessary virtue. We as doctors have all had experiences with patients who cannot be trusted, and I am quite honest with my students about this hard fact of life as a physician. They need to know about the real world if they are going to be on the front lines of primary care medicine.

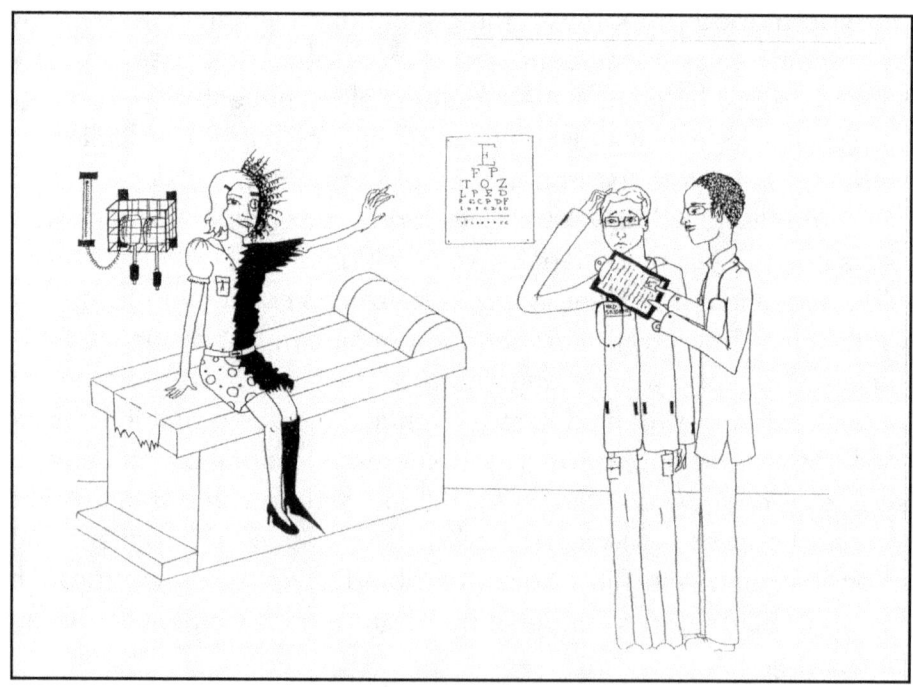

Two sides of the same patient: The Dr. Jekyll/Mr. Hyde scenario.

Case in point is what I call the Dr. Jekyll/Mr. Hyde scenario: Just as the upstanding Dr. Jekyll turned into the monster Mr. Hyde after drinking a potion, so can a patient have a hidden, darker side. For example, the student doctor needs to be aware that it is possible a patient is seeking a prescription for opiates in order to sell them. He may discover that his patient is not telling the truth about his history and is actually drug-seeking. He cannot automatically trust everyone, and needs to act like a detective regarding each patient's true motives for the visit. To illustrate this, I tell the students about James, a 65-year-old man with chronic pain syndrome who had been a patient at the practice for 25 years. This patient was well known to me and his family as a highly reputable and well-to-do member of the community. However, it was discovered that he was taking only two out of the three pills prescribed, and selling the third pill.

I have had a number of eye-opening experiences with this kind of behavior, including a patient who stated that his oxycodone had been flushed down the toilet by his two year old and that he needed another prescription, and another who said her prescription for hydrocodone had been left in New Hampshire at her grandmother's house over the weekend and she needed an early refill. I teach my students that even the most veteran physician who has been in practice for over 30 years can miss this hidden side of a patient. A few years ago, I, along with one of my medical students, treated a former member of the religious community who had moved back to town after a number of years in another state. This man's mother was a fine elderly woman whom I had gotten to know through several house calls. He came to the office complaining of arthritis and chronic pain syndrome and was given prescriptions for antihypertension and diabetes medications and pills for his arthritis. A few days later, the office received five separate phone calls from pharmacies across Connecticut. The patient had apparently written out his own prescriptions for a strong narcotic agent and had signed the doctor's name; it was clear, however, that the prescriptions had been forged, and this supposedly fine, upstanding gentleman landed in prison.

I teach my student doctors that when they enter the examination room they must take a step back and look at the total individual. Most likely what you have in front of you is a very fine person in need of medical care. However, people might have problems you know nothing about. They may have a history of drug abuse or might possibly be in trouble with the law. Impossible as it seems, Mr. Jones might be running a crystal meth factory on the outside. Student doctors must learn to be vigilant. This lesson is an important part of the curriculum.

Sense of Humor

In order to maintain our sanity in the practice of medicine, we need to keep our sense of humor. I truly feel that this helps us in our work as we heal the sick. Every day presents an opportunity to smile. I remember a very impatient elderly patient who demanded in a huff, "What is taking so long?" after waiting only 15 minutes. I gave her a smile and replied, "What do you think this is, a grocery store? We're taking care of sick people here!" My remark helped keep the situation from escalating any further. Another situation that always makes me chuckle is when a patient comes to the office who has carefully researched his problem on the Internet, and has a diagnosis and suggested treatment plan in place. I might jokingly ask him where he got his M.D. degree. And of course, some situations are just plain funny, like the time a student of mine, while performing an ear cleaning, accidentally squirted warm water and peroxide in my face. You've got to laugh. Even though, in truth, we are often dealing with very serious issues all day long, it benefits both the patients and ourselves to keep our sense of humor intact, and this is a lesson the student doctor needs to learn.

CHAPTER 6

Dr. Z.'s Tests and Games

In my 30 years of teaching medical students, I have come to realize that having a student for an approximately four-week rotation is truly too limited. Within that time frame, it is unlikely that each student will be personally exposed to all the various types of patients and medical problems necessary to help her build her knowledge. That is where student tests and games come in: In the Dr. Z. rotation, I use a number of these to reinforce the learning of the student, and any repetition in the cases is intended to help reinforce that knowledge. (Of course, each rotation has a good number of hours dedicated to didactic training of given medical topics, as well as case presentations. My tests are used as an adjunct to these sessions.)

The test questions are constructed in such a way that the students are able to extract the information they need. They are challenged to not only take charge of the total patient and make decisions, right or wrong, regarding his care, but also to consider the psychological, social, and family aspects of the case. I might have each student take on the role of a different consultant (cardiologist, gynecologist, or psychiatrist, for example) for the specific case in question. Even though they may not have completed all of their rotations at this point in their medical training, I feel it is important to let them make decisions and make mistakes, since these mistakes cannot hurt anyone, but will only help their progress. The information they learn can be used in the future to take care of their own real patients. I have included two tests in this book that are representative of the types of questions I might ask. These tests are used to reinforce what the student has or has not learned in the ambulatory care setting.

Question-and-Answer Test

Let's start with the first case given in the test shown in *Figure 2* (Question-and-Answer Test 1). A 59-year-old white male presents with hypertension and diabetes mellitus, type 2. The student will learn from this case how to manage high cholesterol, how to treat diabetes mellitus, why certain medicines can be used in diabetes to prevent complications, and the fact that ACE inhibitors may actually be contraindicated when someone has urticaria. The second question regards a 42-year-old black female who has chest pain, fever, and a cold left foot. Clearly, in this case one is looking for the student's thoughts on the etiology of left foot pain as well as that of a cold left foot. Peripheral artery disease, cerebrovascular disease, thyroid nodules, and atrial fibrillation are certain to be discussed in this case. In the third question, a 90-year-old white female is presenting with weight loss and a right femoral fracture that occurred as she rose from her living room chair. We discuss the problems this patient has with smoking, chronic lung disease, alcoholism, as well as chronic liver disease. Osteoporosis is discussed in detail and preventive medicine is included. The fourth question is asked from the point of view of the student. Your 82-year-old aunt is sitting at the Thanksgiving table; upon finding out you are a medical student, she declares that she is "blind in the left eye." We then discuss the causes of blindness in one eye and possible etiologies. The student is being put on the spot to "act" as a doctor and make decisions. In question 5, I actually throw the student a curveball: List the reasons you want to be a doctor, and discuss how you intend to make a difference in the world. This one provokes many "interesting" answers, as mentioned previously, and I'm always happy when I get something close to the correct Dr. Z. answer: "to help my fellow man."

In question 6, I am simply asking about their basic fund of knowledge: Do they know what defines cardiomyopathy, BOOP syndrome (bronchiolitis obliterans organizing pneumonia), and PIE syndrome (pulmonary infiltration with eosinophilia)? Question 7 asks them to give me the difference between benign monoclonal gammopathy and multiple myeloma. The eighth question, a more general one, concerns a 50-year-old obese white woman who asks, "Why am I always tired?" These types of general questions are very helpful in getting the student to delve deeply into their previous knowledge to come up with "common sense" answers. Question 9 asks for ten causes of headaches that are commonly seen in the ambulatory care setting. A presentation of each type and discussion of how to tell the difference between them using patient history and diagnostic testing is very important. The student doctor is required to know the different causes and will utilize this knowledge in the weeks to come.

Question 10 involves the causes of painful joints in the hands, how one can distinguish between different kinds of arthritis, workups required, and side effects of medications utilized. The next question, number 11, is one of my favorites because it is so often encountered in the primary care setting: Name ten causes of chest pain. I often ask students to name ten or so causes of a certain complaint— it's always helpful to student doctors to have those causes at their fingertips. They may be asking their own medical students the same questions in the future! Question 12 asks for the causes of cough with nonproductive sputum and encourages further discussion of etiology as well as dyspnea on exertion. The student is required to comment on the workup of this patient's palpable left breast nodule, hypertension, diabetes mellitus type 2, hypercholesterolemia, low HDL and very high LDL levels, and increased triglycerides. In this question, GI bleeding and proteinuria are discussed, as well as red blood cell casts and their etiology. Chest X-ray abnormalities such as hilar adenopathy as well as abnormal liver function are introduced. Lastly, question 13 concerns a 35-year-old black female presenting with a 50-pound weight loss in the previous nine months. Discussion of a workup for malabsorption syndrome and other diseases ensues. We also go into the possible results of low B12 levels, and the etiology of malabsorption syndrome, such as viral causes and surgery. Figure 2's Question-and-Answer Test 2 presents 13 additional thought-provoking questions. It is easy to see that these cases have a lot of "meat" in them; however, each question brings something out in the students—when a real-life patient comes to the office with similar complaints, they can utilize the facts learned in the sessions.

Matching Test

In my matching tests (see an example in *Figure* 3), the students are given a list that includes approximately 30 different items on the left side of the sheet to be matched up with a corresponding number on the right. These matching tests contain an extensive amount of information, including what I consider to be "pearls of wisdom" in medicine. Included are syndromes; medications; tumors; general diseases such as diabetes, renal disease, and cardiovascular disease; infectious disease; and allergy phenomena. These topics are intended not only to specifically teach the student to utilize them in the primary care setting, but also for him to think in terms of preventive medicine and proper utilization of medications in the office. They are also designed to be helpful in preparing the students for their board exams. I stress that these diseases and situations are very common in the ambulatory care setting, as well as in hospital cases. Proper reasoning is critical, enabling the student to obtain the correct answers, of course, but more importantly, to make mistakes, which is the best way to learn. This is one of the situations where the beauty of teaching comes in: Their faces light up as they learn, and I can evaluate them on their energy and excitement as they discover the disease processes in medicine.

The matching test also includes treatments of given problems, such as SIADH (syndrome of inappropriate antidiuretic hormone) with a sodium level of 105 and patient seizing, the uses of doxycycline, treatments of TIA (transient ischemic attack), atypical chest pain, breast cancer, the treatment and diagnosis of Hodgkin's disease, diagnosis of insulinoma versus hypoglycemia as reactive etiology, mental status changes, and metabolic disorders. I am always looking for common problems seen in convalescent home patients as well as in house call patients, and this is brought out in the matching questions as well. HIV and its treatment is discussed, although I stress that I am more of a primary care doctor and consultations with the infectious disease specialist are required. Preventive medicine is definitely stressed in these questions; the student is required to know, for example, the preventive medicine required for a female postmenopausal patient as well as for men and women of all ages. Many skin diseases are covered, the more common ones associated with diseases (Reiter's syndrome, ulcerative colitis, insulin-dependent diabetes) as well as those associated with disorders such as polyglandular syndrome and vitiligo associated with Hashimoto's disease and pernicious anemia. Hyperkalemia is another important topic addressed—how to treat it, but also all of its possible causes. This type of question clearly puts the student on the spot in front of five other students, or even in front of me if we are working on a one-to-one basis.

Lab Fest!

Games are an important part of the Dr. Z. rotation. Whether the game involves an individual student or is played in a group setting, they are all helpful in building the students' basic medical knowledge and presenting different ways of handling clinical situations. In a game that I call "Lab Fest," a student is shown a patient's lab data and must give seven causes for each abnormal value. Say a patient's lab work revealed a hematocrit of 20 with an MCV of 120 and TSH of 40. The student might diagnose hypothyroidism and pernicious anemia. He is then required to create a case based on that information, such as a 72-year-old female with dementia and polyglandular syndrome who presents with fatigue and cold intolerance. The student then has to discuss all the causes of anemia and how it is diagnosed, as well as how it relates to hypothyroidism, fatigue, and dementia. Thus, the student is tested on the meaning of the lab data and expands his knowledge of each diagnosis.

Quick Case

In this game, I present 20 quick cases to the students, each consisting of no more than two lines. Examples include an 80-year-old white female presenting with a left temporal headache and blindness (I'm going for mention of temporal arteritis), or a 20-year-old female with slurred speech and hemiparesis (for teaching antiphospholipid syndrome). Each answer makes the student a little smarter.

Rule of Ten

I utilize the Rule of Ten to let students know the importance of having a list of possible etiologies. I simply ask the students, throughout the day, to give me ten causes for a given problem. What are ten causes of hypertension? Ten causes of hyponatremia? Hypotension? What are ten types of headaches and how do you treat them? I use this teaching modality as much as possible throughout the day to provide mental stimulation for the student.

Concept Evolution

I find this exercise to be quite helpful in challenging the student's ability to master the necessary depth of thinking regarding medical topics. I might give an example of a 55-year-old white male who presents to the office with chest pain that has woken him up from sleep. It is pleuritic in nature and associated with a fever of 102 °F. He had a recent cough with yellow sputum production, as well as chills, rigors, and extreme fatigue. He has smoked a pack of cigarettes a day for the last 35 years, has diabetes mellitus, and had been released from the hospital only 10 days previously after sustaining a myocardial infarction. The student is asked to discuss several of the key words mentioned in order to solve this puzzle. For example, regarding the chest pain, what are the possibilities in this case? What are all the causes of chest pain you know? How can you tell the difference between them? If this patient had been diagnosed with pneumonia, I'd ask the student to give me eight causes of pneumonia and tell me how they can be differentiated based on their clinical presentations, with specific symptoms or scenarios. If Legionnaire's disease was the cause of the pneumonia or it was pneumococcal in origin, what organs are involved and what are the clinical presentations? How can you tell the difference between these kinds of pneumonia using the patient's history, physical, and lab data? Regarding the myocardial infarction, give any complications you can think of with MI, such as Dressler's syndrome with pericarditis or ischemic pericarditis. By the way, what causes of pericarditis can you think of? If the student comes back with "rheumatic fever," I'll ask for associations with it, such as the Jones criteria, major and minor.

In the Concept Evolution game, I am gauging the depth of the medical knowledge that each student has obtained. Of course, as the teacher, I am there to fill in any gap in knowledge the student may have. The students find this technique of quickly jumping from one topic to another very stimulating and rewarding in that they are forced to think about things in a challenging way.

Patient Life Game

In one of my favorite games, the students and I invent a patient, and we take that patient through her entire lifetime. It plays out sort of like a soap opera, where the patient's problems, and those of her family, are brought in. With this game, the student is able to see how important it is for her to be aware of the "whole patient," and the whole family unit, in order to institute preventive medicine modalities. I might start with a 25-year-old woman and give her several diagnoses, such as pelvic inflammatory disease, diabetes mellitus, and asthma, and have her experience common exacerbations of each disease, which we discuss. We then move on to the age of 38, when our patient experiences symptoms including muscle weakness and numbness, and is diagnosed with multiple sclerosis. Again, her problems are discussed in detail. At the age of 52, a lump is discovered in her left breast as well as a thyroid nodule. The student must resolve the issue with the appropriate approach including exams, biopsies, ultrasounds, and appropriate consultation. At 62, she has high cholesterol and suffers an unfortunate myocardial infarction. At 72, she has rectal bleeding, which causes weakness and anemia. At 82, our patient suffers a hip fracture while getting up from her kitchen chair, develops colon cancer, and also has peripheral artery disease with neuropathy. Throughout the exercise, important family issues, such as battered woman syndrome, substance abuse, and relatives with Alzheimer's syndrome, might be brought into play. The students are required to discuss preventive medicine for this patient in detail: What health screening techniques could she have had to prevent her medical problems (bone density, HgA1c)? At what age would the student doctor have instituted the proper preventive medicine, for example for diabetes, high cholesterol, colon cancer, and osteoporosis? What could have been done to prevent the myocardial infarction and peripheral artery disease with neuropathy? Which consults could have been called? This game is always fun because the students are challenged to truly think. They are developing their reasoning power and their knowledge of therapeutics. The students feel that they are in charge as they make important decisions regarding our patient.

When designing my tests, I try to include actual real-life situations taken from the lives of my students. The students are thus better able to understand and remember the details. For instance, a student who was recently married in Florida related a situation that had occurred at the wedding involving an elderly person dancing and blacking out. I added this case to one of my matching tests, as well as a situation in which someone had consumed too much alcohol and subsequently experienced electrolyte abnormalities. By doing so, I encourage the students' ability to take situations they have personally experienced and relate them to their own patients. I also like to let the students make up their own cases as a teaching modality. I find it is a great learning tool for them to make up a case of diabetes or high blood pressure and then give the associated medications and side effects.

Every student who has finished the rotation has commented on how helpful these tests are in broadening their horizons and intellectual capacity, giving them a good overview of what can happen to a patient. These kinds of situations, although hypothetical, may help the student tackle future real-life cases. Each student needs to have this background, whether his future is in primary care, family practice, internal medicine, OB/GYN, or psychiatry. The mentor is keying in on the situations of medicine that really cannot be covered in the primary care setting, where a student may only see six or eight patients a day and probably will not have the variety required for proper exposure.

Although I put these tests together for medical students in the ambulatory care setting, they also could be used during any type of hospital rotation. Of primary importance is the student's increased exposure to a variety of problems that may not have been available to him during his rotation. This exposure ensures that the student will fulfill my teaching requirements and fully understand my take-home points. It guarantees that he will secure the required knowledge no matter how busy or unpredictable his office schedule may be during the four to six week rotation. Over the years, I have put together a variety of these tests, and I cannot overstate their importance to the Dr. Z. rotation. I hope the sample tests are useful to readers in building their own versions.

CHAPTER 7

Teaching the Dr. Z. Way

My method of teaching actually begins long before the student even enters my office. It starts with my thought process as I open the official-looking envelope that informs me that a student in his or her third or fourth year of medical training will be arriving soon. At that moment, I have two choices: I can view this student's rotation in my office as a stressful task, or I can regard it as a gift, the gift of helping this man or woman develop into a mature, confident physician. Every time I open one of these envelopes, I know that I am furthering my legacy: to help the students, my patients, and my fellow man.

One of the simplest, and most effective, teaching techniques is to be a good role model. My goal is to get the students motivated and excited about medicine. When they witness my enthusiasm for helping people, it shows them firsthand the beauty of medicine, and they tend to emulate what they see. It is a pleasure to see a student's face light up with excitement and pride when she realizes the joy found in helping others. That is one of the most rewarding moments I experience as a teacher. It is also important that my students understand that I truly enjoy teaching them, and I make sure my actions reflect this. I always notice when progress has been made and make it a point to discuss any skill development in detail with the student. When she makes a mistake, I'll discuss it with her in a constructive way, suggesting a different approach. I accept that the student will make mistakes, knowing that the correction of those mistakes will make her a better total physician. Most importantly, I never degrade the student in any way and always hold her in the highest esteem as a future physician.

Teachable Moments

I take advantage of any teaching moments that may occur during the day. This maximizes the amount of firsthand knowledge the student can learn during a four-week rotation and serves as a wonderful learning mechanism. If my patient presented with left lower quadrant pain and a mass, for example, I would ask the student to come out of the room he was in for a moment, introduce him to the patient as one of my students, and see if he could palpate the mass. I'll have him listen for a patient's positive heart murmur, such as mitral regurgitation or a special gallop rhythm. It is this mechanism of constant learning that enables the student to get the most out of each day in the office. Since it is important that I properly evaluate the student's physical examination methods, I might call a student in to perform a pulmonary exam on a patient of mine with a cough, in order to better evaluate his technique. I also often use the student's previous rotation experience for teaching purposes. I might ask a student with recent experience in psychiatry, for example, to review for me the side effects of medications like tricyclics or benzodiazepines. Perhaps I'd ask a student to discuss malignant neuroleptic syndrome as a cause of rhabdomyolysis with a fever and high CPK. If a student had finished an OB/GYN rotation, the subject might be pelvic inflammatory disease with gonorrhea and Fitz-Hugh-Curtis syndrome.

What Does the Student Think?

Regarding case-based learning in differential diagnosis, my primary objective is to find out what the <u>student</u> thinks is really going on with the patient. I ask open-ended questions like, "What do you think is happening here?" I will not add my own thoughts until I am sure I have gotten everything I can out of him regarding the specifics of his thought process. I ask for specific evidence to back up the student's initial hypothesis, including lab data and history (from a previous visit or recently obtained old records). At that point, I will begin to ask questions about his initial assessment. This is how it works: Say the student is working with a diabetic gentleman who has an HgA1c of 9.7 and is on several medications. I will ask the student, "What do you think is going on with him? Why do you think this patient's HgA1c is so high?" Once I am sure he is on the correct path regarding his thought process, it is time for him to deduce a plan. This patient's diabetes is not under control, so I would ask for his suggestions regarding a change in the medical regimen. Taking into consideration JNC 7 guidelines, what blood pressure should he be looking for in this patient? What type of medications can be used to prevent atherosclerotic events? Again, I always use completely open-ended questions. This is not the time to give answers to the student. If I feel that some teaching needs to take place, I will handle it at the end of the presentation. Thus, each case is a process of deduction and learning.

The student's note-taking process helps him clarify the case in his mind before he presents the case to me. Once he has presented the case and we have gone over the most likely diagnosis, he can complete his note and even expand on it at a later time. Throughout the presentation, I continue to ask, "Why do you think that would be the best idea?" I am aiming to engage the student and challenge him with each patient encounter. I ask tough questions, leading him from one thought to the next, yet try to keep a gentle approach. I try to get the answers out of him no matter how long it takes. If a student said, "I believe this patient is experiencing angina pectoris and that he may be heading for a heart attack," I would not yet tell him my thoughts on the matter. I would ask him why he came to that conclusion; why is that answer more likely than something else? If his thought process seems correct, I will then say, "Very good thinking; I agree with you." The presentation and discussion could take anywhere from 10 to 25 minutes, which might introduce some pressure on the patient flow, but I feel that it is time well spent.

I try never to take the case over from the student. I allow him to truly be in charge of each patient visit. I will also not lecture a student to any degree with a patient in the room. The only time I will interrupt a student is if I feel he is not on the right track; this I do in an open-ended way so as not to totally take over. Rarely, I also might be forced to do so in an unusually busy office setting when there is not enough time to complete each teaching modality.

With this mode of teaching, feedback is on a constant basis. Each patient encounter strengthens the student's diagnostic skills. If his thought process does not seem to be correct, rather than reprimanding him I will suggest other possibilities, allowing him to make his own decisions. I see it as a constant exchange of possibilities and reasoning. I know that every mentor has his or her own teaching techniques. What is important to me is that the student is allowed to be independent in his learning ability. This independence will enable him to gain confidence and reach his true potential.

Minor Office Surgery ━━━━━━━━━━━━━━━━━━━━━━

Another fine adjunct to the practice of teaching medical students in the ambulatory care setting is that of performing minor office surgery. This process really begins with the patient's skin examination. The student is instructed to pay very close attention during the exam, looking at any suspicious skin lesions and marking them down in the office chart. (Drawings are always very helpful.) The student will then discuss with me the possibility of removing any lesions that may be of concern. These lesions may be seborrheic keratosis, basal cell carcinoma, squamous cell carcinoma, or even melanoma. A number of these conditions have been discovered and diagnosed by the medical students who have rotated through my office practice. I stress how important it is to diagnose, and possibly remove, skin lesions before they pose a threat to the patient's health. By performing these procedures herself, utilizing core biopsies for incision and excision, the student can add this experience to her primary office practice. When performing the procedure she is, of course, assisted by me as she begins to learn the technique, or she may utilize her previous experience from another rotation, in surgery perhaps. I find that students are always quite excited about performing office procedures, as well as the potential of utilizing this experience in future office settings. They are actually practicing medicine under close supervision, not merely "shadowing."

Student Requests

What would medical students like to see improved or changed within the primary care teaching setting? I've asked a number of them that question and one thing that always seems to pop up is the desire for more instruction regarding how to perform a focused physical exam and take a focused history. Other comments have dealt with discussion of the specificity and sensitivity of tests and procedures, preventive medicine, and interpretation of lab results and EKG readings. They would like more of a focus on a normal study (a patient with no illness) as opposed to what is present in the disease state. A few students would like more instruction on questioning technique, particularly regarding sensitive issues such as sexual preferences. I keep all of these suggestions in mind as we go through the rotation. Regarding the questioning technique, I have found that it is imperative for the mentor to take the time to help teach the student the art of asking questions, and the best way to talk to the patient about preventive medicine and screening techniques.

CHAPTER **8**

Dr. Z.'s Thirteen-Point Evaluation

Before I begin my evaluation as a judge and coach, at the end of week two, I tell the student my ultimate goal: I am here to help you become the best doctor you can be so you can make a difference in the lives of your patients. (One thing is certain: The so-called halo effect has no place in my practice; that is, whatever the student has done in previous rotations has no bearing on my evaluation.)

I ask myself many questions about the student. Has he truly given the proper amount of energy to each assignment (there is no room for lack of enthusiasm in a busy office)? Has he developed a nice rapport with his assigned patients? Is a high level of independent learning taking place, with the end goal being to further his ultimate knowledge and provide the best differential diagnosis to help each patient (keeping in mind that it is an inescapable fact that students, like all of us, will display weaknesses in knowledge)? The student has gone through a great deal of stress simply fulfilling the requirements of the rotations. As the fledgling physician reaches maturity, he must continue striving toward the ultimate goal of being a student doctor. Soon, I must consider him as a candidate for "ambulatory independent state." The best way of evaluating the student is to closely observe his attitude and diligence during each assigned task. Motivation is a vital component of my evaluation. A willingness to delve into the patient's care to the fullest extent shows the appreciation of medicine and excitement for it that I consider mandatory.

My goal with the thirteen-point evaluation is to use constructive criticism to build confidence and competence in the uncertain student. With this in mind, allow me to present some of the categories that I like to review face to face with the student, namely professionalism, acting ability in the M.D. role, conscientiousness, laboratory data review, telephone calls, office note evaluation, physical exam, history taking, rapport with patients, teaching ability, compassion, developing a differential diagnosis, and finally the student's overall potential as a physician.

Each category receives a grade, usually from A to C. As I tell the students, these grades are not what really matters, but they do provide a gauge of how the student is doing. The comments are what are important for most students, and I make sure they are stated in an honest yet constructive fashion. Let's start with professionalism. Obviously, this means that the student is acting in a professional manner and possesses the demeanor that is appropriate for taking care of patients at the office. He must speak in a professional manner and act like a physician. Next, has the student developed an ability to present himself overall in the M.D. role? Does he give advice in a fashion that is compatible with being a physician, and does he try to act the part? Conscientiousness is almost self-explanatory: Is he conscientious about taking care of his patients and their problems? Is he looking into each specific differential diagnostic possibility and checking that tests have been done in a timely manner? That brings us to lab data review, which entails looking up the laboratory results and checking any further tests. These data could be high glucose, low sodium, low potassium, high cholesterol, or abnormal liver function studies; the student must be checking for abnormal levels and asking me questions about the results. He must also be capable of making decisions regarding specific medications to prescribe following abnormal lab results and regarding further lab testing. Telephone calls should be being made in a timely fashion; these calls will help him establish a rapport with the patient and enable him to show continuity and concern. Office notes are crucial. The history of the present illness, chief complaint, and review of systems must be recorded in a detailed fashion. When we discuss his office notes, I make sure to mention ways that his writing can be improved and give follow-up ideas for each patient. History taking is an important feature. I will observe the student taking a patient history and make sure that he is including pertinent negatives and is able to perform in a directive fashion, noting appropriate details.

At this point in the rotation (during the first two weeks), the student receives constructive criticism on what I've seen thus far regarding his skills during the physical exam. Next, I consider whether the student has been able to develop a good rapport with his assigned patients and has been able to gain their trust. Compassion goes along with this. When a student has compassion, it is clear that he cares about the patient. It is true that there are those individuals who lack this quality, and if that is the case, it's possible that they may actually want to go into pathology or another type of medicine with less patient contact. Compassion, clearly, is difficult to teach, but since I believe most of us went into medicine to help people, it is more a matter of bringing out the compassion that is already there. I will tell a student to try to show more compassion if I feel it is not coming through. A little compassion goes a long way and certainly helps in the patient's overall medical care.

Teaching ability of the patient is a very important skill. Is the student teaching his diabetic patient, for example, about appropriate diet, HbA1c readings, side effects of medication, as well as how cholesterol and blood pressure should be controlled? Procedural ability during surgery performed in the office is also ascertained. Differential diagnosis development is another important category. Any abnormal finding within the history and physical should be designated as a problem, and each problem can have a number of differential diagnoses. For instance, chest pain could result from at least 20 different things, including pleuritis, pneumonia, ischemic heart disease, costochondritis, or pericarditis. Each problem or abnormal finding should prompt the student to consider causes and resolutions.

Finally, I look at the student's overall potential to become a physician. I have seen very few students that I believe really shouldn't have gone into medicine. Although each student's potential varies, in my experience close to 100% of them possess fine potential as physicians as long as they are doing the best they can to seriously study and care for the sick.

Student Reaction

The reactions of the students to this overall evaluation after two weeks of the rotation are usually very positive. They tend to be surprised by the detail in which they are being evaluated. It seems that in most rotations, there is a more general evaluation of the student. However, I find it vital that I truly know the student when I am asked to compose her letter of evaluation for residency. Rather than utilizing a form-type letter, I prefer to give an extremely detailed discussion of each student, noting her positive characteristics and the reasons why I feel she would make an excellent physician. I find that the students are truly excited about being judged as individuals rather than simply as medical students and future doctors.

Two Students: Two Very Different Evaluations

In this section, I detail two student evaluations for comparison purposes. The first student exemplifies very high performance regarding her patient. I will present the case and then outline the steps the student has taken to make a valid differential diagnosis, develop a fine rapport with the patient, handle the differential diagnostic problems, and exemplify many of the characteristics required in order to develop trust in that patient and her family.'

The second illustrative example will be that of a medical student who did not fulfill all of the necessary requirements as a student doctor. I will constructively criticize his performance, and will discuss my reasons for grading him as I did.

First, let's talk about student number 1, a 26 year old named

Mary who previously spent some time doing volunteer work in clinics in India, where she worked with a Mother Theresa group helping the poor. She was asked to handle the following patient: A 63-year-old white female presented to the office with a known history of ischemic heart disease, diabetes mellitus type 2, hypertension, and peripheral vascular disease. The patient was taking metformin, lisinopril (10 mg qd), HCTZ (25 mg po qd), a diabetes-controlling medication (30 mg qd), as well as a sleep medication (10 mg prn). Her history was remarkable for a stroke and breast cancer in her mother, who died at 89, and colon cancer in her father, who died at 58. The patient had been seeing another doctor in California and upon moving to the East Coast was to be followed by my office.

Mary took a very detailed history of present illness and medications. She also took a fine past medical history and surgical history, which included an appendectomy 20 years prior, cholecystectomy 5 years prior, and left ovarian cyst surgery 15 years prior. She determined that the patient had ceased her menstrual cycle at the age of 45. The patient had not been taking supplementation with calcium or vitamin D. A detailed physical exam was performed. Mary was observed to perform the exam in a very orderly fashion using a regional approach that included the 11 organ systems. The findings on the physical exam included diminished pulsation in the left distal extremity as well as a heart murmur, which was consistent with aortic stenosis. Evidence of bilateral retinopathy was also noted. Vital signs were as follows—blood pressure: 140/90, pulse: 70, respiratory rate: 15, and no fever. Also noted were nicotine stains on most of the digits of the patient, who was a 1½-pack-a-day smoker for 40 years. The laboratory tests ordered by Mary included blood sugar, lipid profile, electrolytes, urine, EKG, echocardiogram, and chest X-ray. She also ordered a pulmonary function study and told the patient to return in one week so they could discuss the laboratory results. Mary advised the patient regarding preventive medicine, such as the need for a colonoscopy because her father had died of colon cancer, as well as mammography, bone density, and smoking cessation. She advised the patient regarding tests for peripheral disease and recommended that she visit an ophthalmologist, podiatrist, and cardiologist for a workup. She asked the appropriate questions for peripheral artery disease as well as for ischemic heart disease. A week later, the patient returned and stated that Mary had indeed called her two days after the office visit, showing concern for her problems and asking how she was doing with the medications prescribed (Mary had increased the lisinopril to 20 mg since the blood pressure was elevated). On the follow-up visit, she counseled the patient regarding acceptable levels of important parameters: She told her to have an HbA1c every three months, and to strive for an LDL under 70 and HDL over 60. She counseled her on smoking cessation, showing support and concern. Mary also found out that the patient was a victim of domestic violence, which was the reason she had left California; her husband had inflicted bodily injury as well as emotional abuse for many years. After the second visit, Mary called her again to see how she was doing emotionally and to counsel her on possible local community domestic violence support.

On Mary's evaluation, I noted that she certainly showed a fine rapport with the patient, did a very good job regarding differential diagnosis, and also revealed a high degree of professionalism in the way she handled the patient. She was conscientious about the lab data and about the patient's problems. Her lab data review was excellent in that she asked me about abnormal lab data and how to handle them. We also discussed which medications she could use (she suggested a statin), and she went over possible side effects with the patient. Mary was clearly developing a good differential diagnosis; if she did not know a detail or a fact, she would take the time to look it up to further her knowledge. Her physical exam and history taking were quite adequate, and her rapport with the patient was excellent, as evidenced by the patient calling the student several times over the next few weeks regarding her medication. Her teaching ability was also fine—she taught the patient what she should be doing to prevent further complications from diabetes, including atherosclerosis, retinopathy, renal disease, and heart disease. I complimented Mary on her compassion toward this patient, especially after it was revealed that she was a battered woman. I noted that her overall potential as a physician was very high.

Next, let's consider student number 2, Ben, a 26 year old from Louisiana. His case concerns a 77-year-old white female with a history of abdominal pain, ischemic heart disease, myocardial infarction, and a cardiac catheterization that had been performed about six months prior due to a 60% blockage in the left anterior descending artery. The patient had hypertensive heart disease, high cholesterol, and was obese; she experienced severe abdominal pain during the visit and seemed quite fearful—Ben was very concerned about this patient. The exam findings were as follows: essentially normal vital signs, she was not jaundiced or cyanotic, regular heart rhythm, a 2/6 systolic murmur, lungs clear, and diffuse abdominal tenderness in the epigastric region, left lower quadrant, right lower quadrant, and left upper quadrant. There was a negative Murphy's sign. The patient rated the pain after eating as a 7 out of 10, stating that it radiated down over the whole abdomen to the point of excruciating discomfort. Ben asked the patient to return in a week, after my suggestion. He ordered lab work, but failed to check on the results, although he did call her later in the week to see how she was doing. He also did not find the time to review the patient's laboratory data or CT scan. Rather, he came in and began seeing other patients without asking about or reviewing this patient's lab work; he reviewed it after the patient returned to the office a week later. The patient's workup was thorough, including laboratory data consisting of CBC (normal), electrolytes (normal), and renal function (normal), and she did see a gastroenterologist. When she came in the following week, the pain had actually increased and she was admitted to the hospital. It was not clear what the problem was, but possibilities included ischemic bowel disease or mesenteric ischemia (the patient was eventually diagnosed with mesenteric ischemia and renal artery stenosis). Ben did show compassion for the patient, and he visited the hospital the day she was admitted and talked to her in detail about diagnostic possibilities. The patient and Ben developed an excellent rapport and she called him several times to discuss her case; however, overall he should have displayed more interest in checking her lab data and CT scan, as well as her condition the day after being sent home from the office. He also could have asked more questions regarding other diagnostic possibilities. Overall, Ben received a high grade for his rapport and compassion for this patient. However, his laboratory review was inadequate and he was therefore given a B– in that regard. His conscientiousness was not up to par, nor was his teaching ability regarding subsequent visits to address such concerns as hypertension and obesity. He did act in a quite professional manner in the role of physician, but he didn't do well with his telephone calls. His office notes were rated as adequate, and he was instructed on how to improve them by further developing the history of the patient's present illness and expanding on his thoughts regarding differential diagnosis with pertinent negatives.

These examples provide a framework that helps us view the students and assess their needs. What is most important is that the student is doing his best and showing energy, compassion, conscientiousness, and independent learning. Skill in differential diagnosis will certainly expand with time. A student who has had only a few rotations prior to entering an outpatient setting cannot be expected to give a differential diagnosis of seven problems. However, he at least should be expected to know how to view abnormal laboratory data and abnormal physical findings and how to take an adequate history. I admit it is not easy in a four-week rotation to truly uncover every quality of every student and assess his true potential as a physician. This ability depends a great deal on how much time the mentor is prepared to spend reviewing the student's performance with him. Every mentor will have a different idea of what makes a good student doctor; however, the most important task for each mentor is to spend a good amount of time with the student, and show concern for him, making him realize that this constructive criticism will result in an evaluation that can be used to make him a fine M.D. He needs to know that your goal is to make him a total physician, one who will care about the emotional, physical, and psychological concerns, including the family dynamics, of each patient.

It is now time to allow the student to graduate from the first two weeks of the rotation and move on to the second section, the automatic pilot phase. Although the students know that I am always available to help them, they are given more independence than they had in the first two weeks.

CHAPTER 9

Student Independence Day

At the end of the second week, after the student doctor has received her thirteen-point evaluation, I let her know that she is now on automatic pilot. By this time, she should have enough basic knowledge to go into each room, make her own assessment after a careful history and physical exam, and decide on specific testing, medication, and a future plan for each patient, including screening suggestions and when to return to the office for follow-up. The student's new sense of independence seems to give a boost to her energy level. By now she feels more comfortable in the role of the student doctor and is much less intimidated by the patient. She is diving into the patient's problem at a much higher level.

Developing a Differential Diagnosis

It is important for each student to have enough confidence that they can present me with the differential diagnosis I would expect at this stage. They should be starting to narrow their focus on a specific symptom at this point, beginning to pinpoint what is wrong with the patient. After leaving the room, the student should have a reasonable hypothesis with supporting data and be able to give me a case presentation that is brief and to the point yet provides enough information that I can comment on the student's thoughts regarding his differential diagnosis.

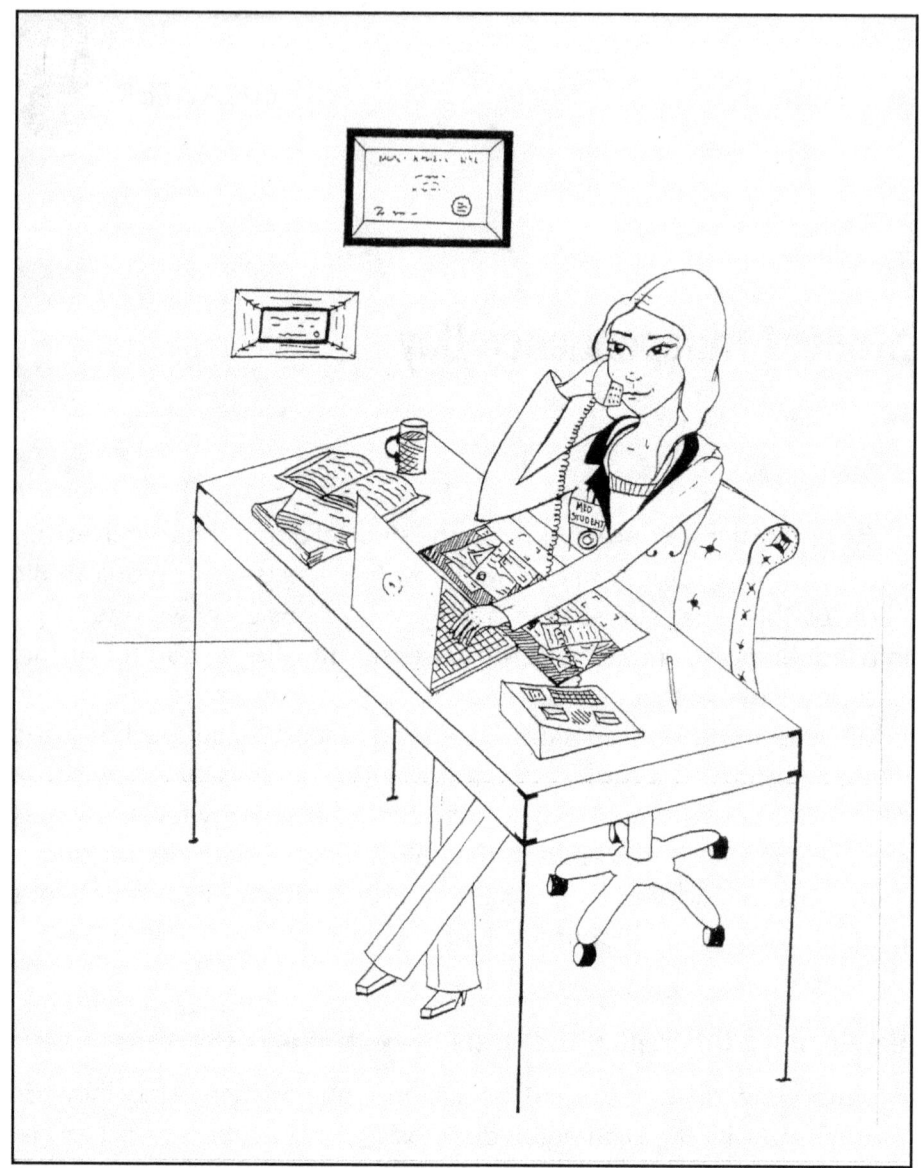

The multitasking med student.

Say the student leaves the room and presents the case to me, giving a differential diagnosis of hyponatremia. He should have a good idea of the causes of hyponatremia, and if he doesn't, we will go over the information quickly at that time and discuss it further later. If a patient presents with right upper quadrant pain, and the student gives a differential diagnosis of pancreatitis or peptic ulcer disease, for example, I will ask him how he came to that conclusion. If I am not satisfied with the response, I will ask him open-ended questions in order to deduce his reasoning, and I will correct him as we go along. If a student mentioned that he thought peptic ulcer disease was a good possibility with a patient with left upper quadrant pain, I would ask him to tell me the ways peptic ulcer disease usually presents, its relieving factors, and ask him to list likely possibilities. There is never a definite end, in other words, to differential diagnosis discussion. The student is required to go home each day and look into other differential diagnostic possibilities for each patient. This helps him begin to see the truth behind the "50% rule" (for the patient's first visit, he probably will only be able to diagnose the problem half the time). It is vital that the student not be overconfident, and understands that his knowledge will grow with every differential diagnosis he presents to me.

Students will continue to gain confidence during the automatic pilot segment of the rotation. They need to be able to go from room 1, with a patient who has abdominal pain, for example, to room 2, with a patient experiencing chest pain, and order proper testing for each one. And all of this is expected to be done within 15 minutes or so for each patient! Seeing more than one patient at a time is possible, but certainly not easy, and can probably only be learned after many years of primary care and ambulatory care practice.

Preventive Care

I make very clear to my students the importance of teaching preventive care to the patient. The student doctor needs to understand the disease process in order to teach proper preventive care. Using her own words, in layman's terms, she can teach the patient in a way he can truly understand what problems he might be likely to face in the future. Let's use the example of a 54-year-old patient with diabetes mellitus and hypercholesterolemia. The student would review what high cholesterol is, its potential complications, and the goals we as physicians have in dealing with diabetes mellitus. She would bring up LDL and HDL, as well as atherosclerosis and its overall effects on the body. She would discuss which medications were being chosen for this patient and why, including their value in prevention of renal disease in diabetes, such as effect on efferent arteriolar pressure. The student becomes a true teacher to her patient. She is the authority in the examining room at that moment.

Competence Gained

Throughout weeks three and four, the weekly three-hour session continues to take place, and I continually present the students with problems to solve in order to complement their clinical acumen (such as asking them to give me ten causes of hypercalcemia). When they order tests, I ask them to tell me what knowledge can be gained from each one. Thus, I can be sure that their basic knowledge is in place at this stage of the rotation, that they know, for example, that blood pressure in a diabetic patient should be 130/80 or lower and LDL cholesterol should be less than 70.

I'd like to stress that the independence of the student is the hallmark of the third and fourth week. I tell the student that she is truly in charge of her patients. She will have control over the ordering and evaluation of patient tests. If a chest X-ray has been ordered in a smoker and a lung lesion is found, or a thyroid lesion is found on an ultrasound test, the student is required to tell me what she wants to do and how she is going to do it. Obviously, if the student is not on the right track, I will guide her in her decision-making process.

There are many rewarding moments for the student doctor at this point in the rotation: The look of relief on a patient's face when bloodwork shows that the statin she suggested has brought down the cholesterol level. Knowing she has contributed to saving a life by suggesting a preventive procedure such as colonoscopy or mammography. The moment when a patient with depression or a seemingly insurmountable family problem such as domestic violence realizes that someone can help them. As a teaching physician, there is much that I find gratifying at this stage of the rotation as well: The student is functioning independently in many ways. She is showing responsibility and truly taking care of her patients. When I tell the student that by her very presence in the room, she is a part of the healing process for the patient, and I see her face glow, I feel a deep sense of satisfaction.

At the end of each day, time permitting, I like to talk to each student to see if there's any topic he'd like to learn more about, and to ascertain how comfortable (or uncomfortable) he feels in the examining room. When a student tells me truthfully what is on his mind, I can adjust my teaching practices for his individual needs. If a student is trying very hard, for instance, yet he feels he is not quite ready for the automatic pilot phase, I will be there to get him through this at every level of his development. In the automatic pilot phase, the student suddenly becomes a "doctor" in my office. The pressure is on as he is required to go into the examining room to talk to the patient and perform a physical, come out of the room with a carefully gathered history and evaluation of the chief complaint, and present me with a useful differential diagnosis and plan of attack. One thing is certain at this stage: The student must be able to make a useful differential diagnosis treatment plan. He must follow up after that patient so he is aware of the effects of the treatment. He must call the patient, and check laboratory and X-ray results when appropriate. He is truly taking over the case. I find this to be a very exciting time because I can actually see what I've taught him coming to fruition. I watch the students' expressions when they learn something about the art of being a physician, and for me that is the ultimate thrill of teaching.

CHAPTER 10

Evolution of the Student

Under the Mentor's Wing

The student's level of independence is the primary difference between the first two weeks of the rotation versus the second two weeks. In the first half of the rotation, a visit might go something like this: Our patient, Mr. Adams, is a 72-year-old white male with diabetes mellitus, hypertension, and peripheral neuropathy. He is suffering from sexual dysfunction and nocturia (three times per night). He is taking metformin, another diabetes medication, a cholesterol-lowering medication, aspirin, and an antihypertensive. His history included his father's death from colon cancer. The student, Lee, has done a focused exam, checking blood pressure, diabetes mellitus follow-up, peripheral artery disease, and cardiovascular disease including the heart and carotid artery. Lee has presented the case to me, and we have gone back into the examining room together.

"Good morning, Mr. Adams," I say. "Lee has told me you are taking your medications on a regular basis, checking your sugar, and he says that your blood pressure is running 140 over 96, your pulse is 75, and you are having to get up at night several times to use the bathroom as well as having some sexual difficulty." I inform Mr. Adams that I will be checking him as well, and I go on to perform a focused exam, demonstrating to the student how I would check the heart, lungs, and abdomen, and how I would do a peripheral vascular exam. My goal here, during the first two weeks of the rotation, is to be a role model for the student. I want him to see that I truly enjoy taking care of Mr. Adams. I have developed a strong rapport with him over the years and, I hope, have demonstrated professionalism, class, caring, and compassion. Those are qualities I want Lee to see in me as I work with the patient. As the visit goes on, after he has given me his complete plan, I indicate to Lee my additional suggestions on how to follow a patient with diabetes mellitus, including the goal of the HgA1c and the various cholesterol parameters that are needed, such as LDL, HDL, total cholesterol, and triglycerides. I go over necessary testing like cardiac CRP, homocysteine, and of course colon cancer screening. I review possible sexual dysfunction etiologies, including diabetes and/ or hypertension. We discuss whether this patient needs a prostate exam, PSA, or yearly EKG, and in general go over any screening possibilities for a patient of this age, including testosterone level.

All this time, it is clear that Lee has been watching me closely. He is seeing how a doctor who has been in practice for many years is handling a patient's multiple problems, and at the same time trying to develop that patient's sense of trust and comfort. I make sure the excitement I feel in caring for this patient is evident to Lee. My goal is to show the student that there is a beauty in taking care of one's fellow man. It may turn out that Lee is not interested in primary care medicine or family practice in the ambulatory setting; however, he will always remember what it was like to be a physician in this capacity in the early 21st century, and he can apply this knowledge to any field he chooses.

The Student Takes the Reins

Now we are in the second half of the rotation: the automatic pilot stage. It is the follow-up visit of Mr. Adams. Again, Lee presents the case to me. This time, however, since Mr. Adams is now

Lee's patient, I would ask, "What are your plans for future care, such as screenings and Mr. Adams's diabetes and hypertension regimens?" Lee goes over the diabetes regimen and tells me how he will monitor the patient's HgA1c, cholesterol (aiming to get his LDL below 70 and his HDL over 65). He goes over his plans for hypertension management, which include an ACE inhibitor to bring the blood pressure at or below 130/80, per JNC 7 guidelines. He states that he will monitor Mr. Adams's EKG and cardiac state once a year, and will call special consultation as necessary. He will recommend a screening colonoscopy. He will monitor the patient's feet for calluses and fungal infections and will recommend that he see a podiatrist every 1–2 years, an ophthalmologist yearly, and be monitored by a cardiologist. He will also monitor the patient for the potential of peripheral artery disease. It is clear that Lee is striving to present a picture of total care for his patient. I ask him what he is recommending for lab work (mentioning that parameters such as cardiac CRP and homocysteine need to be monitored) and we might discuss medication side effects and possible damaging interactions.

At this point, I inquire about his plans for teaching preventive medicine to the patient (I may observe him as he does so). I want him to become a student teacher as well as a student physician. This teaching needs to be done in his own words, so that he can establish a rapport with the patient. Such a rapport will make it easier for the student to call the patient later on the phone if a problem shows up on the lab work, or simply to see how the patient is doing. By stepping back, I am showing the student that he is in charge. Of course, I am standing on the sideline closely observing his techniques and discussion on the phone and will intervene if needed. By this time, in the third and fourth week, the student has evolved and is growing into the M.D. role. He is well equipped to make a difference in society, and I am proud to have been a part of it.

CHAPTER 11

A Successful Patient Encounter

There are many variables that contribute to a successful patient encounter. For the student, the patient visit is an exciting yet extremely complicated situation. One of the first things she can do to make it a little easier is to know which type of visit she is dealing with. Is it a brief 5–10 minute visit, like a blood pressure check? An intermediate or extended visit, which may entail taking into consideration two or even up to five problems? A complete physical? Each of these types of visits will involve varying levels of discussion with the patient and a different approach to the exam. For example, for a brief office visit, a review of systems may not be necessary; perhaps only the vital signs need to be taken or a heart or lung exam, depending on the complaint. An extended visit might require examination of as many as four or five systems. If she has an idea ahead of time of how she will handle that patient, it makes it much easier for her to complete her assignment and present the case to her teaching attending.

It is vital that the student be as relaxed as possible as she enters the room. To help ensure that that is the case, prior to the visit I will have given her any patient information I feel might be helpful, such as any medications he might be on, or what has happened to him in the last few months, such as being in the hospital or having syncope or chest pain. I will frame each expectation that I have for the student, so she can limit her time in the room and not be looking for extraneous facts that really do not have much consequence regarding the patient's chief complaint.

A successful patient encounter might play out as follows: The medical student, after entering the room and introducing herself, might shake the patient's hand in a cordial fashion, thereby beginning to establish a rapport with him. Especially on a first visit with a patient, I advise the student to take a few moments getting to know the patient, and perhaps asking about his family. As mentioned previously, it's nice to be able to ask a returning patient about something that was discussed in a previous visit, such as inquiring about his trip to Florida. Per my suggestion, the student doctor speaks slowly and somewhat softly to help the patient relax. She allows the patient to give his history for at least 5 minutes, while taking notes for accuracy. She can then start directing the patient to her agenda for the patient visit. I teach the student that a strong history of present illness represents the possible differential diagnosis.

While she begins to ask the patient questions, including of course pertinent medical history and habits, she starts the examination using an organized technique. Although she has been taught that performing exams regionally and pointed toward the chief complaint is vital in a busy medical office, she is also aware that the physical exam represents only about 15% of the total when deciding on the differential diagnosis and treatment plan. A minimal exam would include vital signs; head, eyes, ears, nose, and throat; and cardiac, pulmonary, and peripheral vascular exams. She performs a focused exam depending on the complaint.

As the patient becomes more relaxed, it is important to follow a specific format to bring out the appropriate diagnoses. She asks the patient appropriate pointed questions to delineate the possibilities that she will utilize in her differential diagnosis and treatment. Thus far, the student has probably spent about 12 minutes in the room. Keeping in mind time constraints, she slowly begins backing out of the room, saying she wants to discuss the case with Dr. Z. and will be back. She continues to speak softly and in a kind fashion. No matter what the problem entails, I always want the student to show compassion and kindness. She is encouraged to never forget the importance of social and psychological issues, and to take charge of those issues, since they may be more challenging than the medical aspects of the case. For instance, a 44-year-old patient who recently lost his mother may require a much more extensive visit to help him cope with his loss.

As the student presents the case to me, she clearly relates her thoughts regarding the history of present illness and gives me a potential group of diagnostic possibilities. She knows that any abnormal findings in the history or physical exam need to be resolved or at least noted. She demonstrates a good thought process involving the accurate assessment of each problem and potential resolution and treatment plan.

We reenter the room together and I take any further history and try to bring out the important features that will help guide the student to making the best diagnosis. If there are other findings that I think are pertinent, such as a herpes zoster rash or a significant heart murmur, I interrupt the student in a professional fashion and reveal the information. I always ask the student what she thinks. This enables the student to realize that I regard her thoughts as important, and instills confidence in her, so she is better able to reason out her differential diagnostic possibilities. Remember that the attending physician is the student's model. Each student will require a different amount of time and different degree of attention, and it is the mentor's job to bring out the best in each one.

In the last 5 minutes of the visit, the student performs the important patient teaching, being sure to discuss side effects of medications, drug interactions, and overall plans that we have discussed. As necessary, she uses her own teaching skills to educate the patient on topics such as hypertension, diabetes mellitus, headaches, chest pain, and shortness of breath. She understands that preventive medicine teaching is vital.

Finally, the student doctor makes sure she will be available for that patient's follow-up visit if possible, so she can continue to be a part of this patient's care.

It takes much practice and persistence to succeed in developing a more extensive and successful patient encounter. There are many challenges in a busy primary care practice, but as the student doctor discovers her strengths, she will grow into a strong healer. A vital part of this growth is a strong mentor–student relationship that is based on trust and the excitement of learning. We are learning from each other every day. The jungle of the office setting with all its difficult characters and complexities is now becoming an exciting world for the student. She is starting to possess the proper tools and knowledge necessary to handle today's complicated medical system. With each day she becomes more confident and utilizes her time more effectively and productively.

CHAPTER **12**

The Doctor–Patient Relationship

Let's focus on the relationship between the doctor (and this obviously includes the student doctor) and the patient. Is the relationship alive or dying? It has certainly suffered in the last 20 years, due in part to pressures from the HMOs with their constant scrutiny of the physician's decisions, second opinion required on almost any diagnosis, preauthorization of medications, and the need for adequate note taking and risk management. All of these requirements make it extremely difficult for the ambulatory care physician to spend the necessary time with each patient. However, it is vital that the physician, and the student physician, develop a familiar, trusting relationship with his patients. Remember Marcus Welby, with his kind, warm bedside manner? That kind of doctor is invaluable to his patients. Patients frequently feel like just a number. They want to feel that the doctor knows them and has the time to spend to talk to them as people.

It is true that some health-care professionals, including busy physicians in the ambulatory setting, can succumb to the pressure. The modern physician might seem to be detached from his patients, appearing somewhat rigid and distant. He might appear to be a one-dimensional, robotic machine as he goes through the day. Maybe he seems like a bull in the ring, with the patient as the matador. This doesn't have to be the case. Working on the front lines, as a vital part of the health-care team, the student doctor can strive to be a warm, sincere, and compassionate listener who is truly excited about helping to solve the problems in his patients' lives. He can discover their special, individual qualities while gaining the trust required to help them. One way for the student doctor to find a little extra time to spend with the patient is for him to ask the patient to jot down a list of questions and concerns prior to the follow-up visit, as well as symptoms and medications, including herbal preparations and vitamins, or even to bring the bottles with him. This may improve efficiency in the shortened time available within a busy schedule, and encourages the student and patient to relate to each other more effectively.

What was our goal when we entered the medical profession? It certainly wasn't to become a cold, noncommunicative, troubled soul. The student can become more like the doctor of old by striving to bring less pressure into the ambulatory care setting. Patients should feel comfortable enough to ask important questions regarding their care. In order to improve rapport with the patient, the student is taught to be concise and to phrase his evaluation and treatment in a way that the patient can easily understand. Having a family member present may also mediate the concerns of patients who may not understand what the physician or student doctor is saying.

A Small-Town Physician and Mentor

In my early days as a physician, I worked with a wonderful doctor named Dr. Jack Galen, who had been a small-town family physician for over 45 years. (It is a wonderful lesson in continuity of care when students realize that some of my patients have actually been a part of the practice for longer than I have been!) Dr. Galen was a total family doctor: He made house calls (as I do), delivered babies, performed appendectomies, and assisted in many complicated surgical procedures at the local hospital. He taught me to enter the examining room in a calm fashion and to try to be very familiar with each patient. He told me to smile and to speak softly, and to leave the room by slowly backing away. Of course, he also knew the importance of taking an adequate history as well as performing a focused physical exam. In turn, as part of my mentoring of the student doctors who rotate in my practice, I teach them to speak softly and slowly, to listen to the patient's history for 5–10 minutes, then take over the discussion in a directive fashion, and begin to make their way out of the room within about 15 minutes (for an intermediate exam). The staff can do testing, lab work, EKGs, and schedule X-rays if necessary after the student leaves the room for the first time and presents the case to me. She can return to the examining room later to discuss her plans for the patient, including her thoughts on what to teach the patient about preventive medicine. I train the student to plan her time in the examining room in a constructive manner. By doing so, she can more easily deal with the high-pressure reality of modern ambulatory medicine in the busy and often unpredictable office setting.

We are living in a modern world, but within this world there is still a place for the old-fashioned family doctor like Marcus Welby and Jack Galen. Let's bring back that kind of doctor. Let's teach compassion, rapport, and patient education, all of which are sorely missed in the high-tech systems of modern medicine. The complicated environment in which we function today can also incorporate wonderful rapport and conscientiousness regarding the problems of each patient. We can have the kindness and the beauty of medicine just like it used to be in the early days. The 21st century can have the family doctor back.

CHAPTER **13**

Student Concerns

"I Only Want to See Dr. Z."

There are a few hurdles that tend to pop up with regularity during the rotation. One of these is what I call the "I only want to see Dr. Z." syndrome. There are many reasons why a patient might feel reluctant to see the student doctor. They may feel that it is a burden to provide the student with their whole medical history, and feel more comfortable with someone who already knows their case. Maybe they simply feel awkward dealing with someone they are not familiar with. This situation could have the unfortunate result of the patient not divulging important medical information, whether due to embarrassment because the student is unfamiliar to him or because the patient has trouble bonding with someone he might only see once. For whatever reason, the patient may not want to be a learning tool.

How can the teaching physician help break the ice? I find it useful to present the student as an important member of the health-care team who is helping me with that patient's care, rather than simply as a student. I learned this from my mentor, Dr. Galen. Back when I was a new physician, Dr. Galen would always present me to patients as a fine individual who knew the patient's case and would perform in their best interests. This helped establish the patient's trust in me, and this trust also allowed me to take over that patient's case when Dr. Galen retired. When I first bring a student with me into the examining room, I might say, "Hi Ms. Smith, this is Jack, who is a medical student from Yale, and he's going to help me with your case today." I'll go on to say something positive about him such as, "He's a fine student who would like to ask you some questions." Before I leave the room, I mention that I will be returning soon. By introducing the student to the patient, I find the patient tends to be more relaxed about the encounter and is usually quite cooperative about seeing the student. If the patient has been seen at the office previously, the student is taught to establish some familiarity with him by asking how he is doing with his previous problems: "How have your headaches been since your last visit?" if he had been having migraines, or "How is your sugar being controlled?" for a patient with diabetes. Prior to the student entering the examining room, I have given him a synopsis of the patient, including any pertinent history such as hypertension, diabetes, cancer, or psychological issues. The student reads any previous notes as well. The more the student knows about the patient, the better.

If the student is on his own, he might say, "Hi, I'm Jack Brown. I'm a student from Yale who's working with Dr. Zaretzky. I'll be going over your tests with you." This is part of the acting role, mentioned previously; the student is acting the part of the doctor, and the more he does so, the more comfortable he'll feel in the role. Consulting the chart, he might go on to say, "I understand you were seen for a cough on the last visit. How is that?" If there is a notation in the chart that the patient had been looking forward to her daughter's wedding, for instance, the student doctor might go on to ask how everything went. Again, this helps to break the ice and place the patient (and possibly her family if they are also in the room) at ease.

I once received a letter from a patient who initially felt wary about seeing a student doctor, but ended up changing his mind. I think it gives some insight into how a patient might be feeling in that situation. He wrote: "After having a doctor for almost a decade who knows 'everything' about you, it is hard to be approached by a medical student who only knows you from a medical chart and brief history. There are some ailments that I think I wouldn't bring up to a student. I wonder if this is because I don't know this person, or am I worried that it will take forever if I start telling him the whole nine yards? I finally realized that by seeing the student I am helping him with his medical growth. It is his job to learn and absorb everything he can. I do try to keep my answers as brief as possible and straight to the point so the student can make his diagnosis and treatment. Although there will never be a doctor like my doctor, I feel comfortable with the student because I know he is being taught by the best—that's right, the best." Signed D.B., 2/1/07.

Time Constraints

Students feel quite a bit of pressure from the time constraints in the office, especially when they catch sight of a busy waiting room. They feel that if they spend too much time in the room they will upset the office flow, but if they spend too little time they will miss pertinent information. And it is true at this point that some students may be very gradual in their work, making patient flow extremely difficult. (Also, at this stage of their training, some students feel they can't "escape" from the room if the patient continues to talk.) As a primary care doctor, I am well aware myself of the pressure resulting from time constraints. To help ease this feeling in my students, I try to teach them how to work in an efficient manner so as to enhance adequate patient flow, yet I always stress that time is not the most important thing, and if necessary the patient can always return for a follow-up visit. In fact, I make sure to give the students at least one day in which they are required to see about a dozen patients. This helps bring home the fact that they may not be able to obtain every bit of information they need on one visit, and another visit might be necessary to make the final diagnosis.

Note Taking

Another common concern a student might have is whether she is taking adequate notes. Although, of course, as mentioned previously, I teach proper note-taking technique, I am also sure to reassure the student that she can always reschedule the patient or call him, and that she will get a second, third, or fourth crack at the history after the assigned visit. It is true that progress notes have to be very detailed and appropriately written to satisfy insurance requirements, such as Medicare. The student frequently will need to finish her thought process after the patient visit. To make sure these thoughts are fresh, I encourage students to complete their notes on the same day as the visit. I review the notes in detail and offer comments. As the rotation goes on, the students' notes start to evolve from brief and general to more detailed and meaningful.

Feelings of Inadequacy

Students are learning every day, yet may still feel incompetent regarding how they are taking care of patients. They may feel that their knowledge of certain topics or illnesses is inadequate. I reassure students that it takes a great deal of experience, as well as study and research, to possess the tools needed to practice the art of medicine. An outgrowth of this feeling of inadequacy is the concern that their diagnostic skills are somehow lacking. They worry that they aren't examining the correct body system(s) regarding the present illness, as well as noting pertinent negatives. I tell them that at this point in their careers, they shouldn't worry too much about their differential diagnostic skills. They will need years of practice before they will be completely comfortable with patient diagnosis.

CHAPTER 14

Office Surprises

Student doctors need to be prepared that there are "unexpected surprises" that occasionally occur in ambulatory care. Case in point: One of my students had a 48-year-old male patient who had come to the office because of a headache. After determining that this seemed to be a tension headache, the student asked what was he so "tense" about. He was trying to get some information on the patient's family background and any possible dynamics that might have been contributing to the problem. The student listened carefully, since as we all know, listening is a very important part of a medical visit. The patient stated that the problem was his wife: They hadn't had good sexual relations for over 10 years. The student asked why that was and was told, "Because my life is being controlled by the gorillas and orangutans at the Bronx Zoo." The patient went on to say that the animals were the "jungle authority" and they had told him to stay away from his wife sexually. He said the jungle authority was involved in an antifascism movement around the world, and the head of the jungle authority and chief executive officer was named Andy. The student told me later that he was so surprised by this dialogue that his first reaction, in all honesty, had been to chuckle inside. The student was well aware, however, that this patient needed to be handled with a great deal of compassion; he had a serious problem and needed an immediate psychiatric consult. It turned out that the patient's psychiatric medications needed to be adjusted and, after some in-hospital care, he was able to be managed on an outpatient basis. The lesson here for the student doctor is to be prepared for anything!

CHAPTER 15

Outside Teaching Venues

The Nursing Home

As a primary care physician, I find it important to follow my patients when they can no longer perform their activities of daily living and must enter a nursing home. It is quite helpful to have the ambulatory medical student accompany me to evaluate these patients. Not only do I think it is an excellent teaching tool because of the numerous medical issues that arise, but tapping into the compassion of the medical student can awaken his ability to see the beauty of taking care of the many charming elderly residents of convalescent homes.

Each elderly person possesses a unique history of life. Whether they came from another country and have intriguing cultural differences, or are just interesting people, I feel there is actually a special "cuteness" about them, and being able to recognize this beauty is an important part of nursing home care. When the student converses with the patient while he obtains her history, he also learns about the patient's history of life, and begins to understand how important the end of life can be. He starts to comprehend the sense of comfort he is bringing to the nursing home resident as he cares for her, and the soothing sense of connection to another human being that an elderly person might feel when anyone stops to talk to her.

It is important for the student to understand the complexity of geriatric medicine. Members of this age group are often on multiple medications that can produce a vast array of interactions and side effects. They may have many unusual physical findings that can add to the wealth of the student's knowledge. Within this unique educational setting, the student will also learn about the various state regulations and requirements for the physician.

In a nursing home visit, after the history and physical are completed by the student, he presents the case to me and any other medical students present. We discuss medical issues that arise on a monthly, weekly, or daily basis. This enables the student to understand the evolution of a patient's care from the office setting to the convalescent home for chronic care. The students are asked what they can do to help these patients. Although the answers to that question are quite diversified, it is important for the student to realize that his presence, with care and compassion, will make that geriatric patient feel better. The students learn that isolation, hearing deficit, and losing one's abilities to function can cause depression. In the elderly, even low dosages of certain medications can cause many manifestations of changing mental status. A good deal of psychiatry can be taught here in trying to understand how and why different medications are utilized. These medications can include antidepressants, atypical antipsychotics, and many medications used for agitation and insomnia. Throughout my nursing home teaching, it is my hope that the student understands he has the power to improve the quality of life for our elderly treasures, who are oftentimes forgotten.

House Calls

The house call has always been a wonderful modality of teaching for me, as the students learn how diverse and satisfying this experience can be. On a house call to visit a 40-year-old woman with multiple sclerosis, my students were able to witness how difficult it is for some patients to cope with their disease. This patient was so severely debilitated that she was unable to use her contracted legs to walk and had to resort to using her hands to move around the living room. They saw the patient utilizing bee venom from actual beestings as an adjunctive therapy (the patient was stung six times per day), and learned that she had done so for many years since it afforded her several hours of relief from her symptoms each day. (The patient's husband provided the venom from his beehives.) This patient's bravery and open-minded attitude toward her disease were an inspiration to the students.

On a house call to visit a 94-year-old patient with atherosclerosis, ischemic heart disease, and hypertension, a student arrived at the house to find her in the kitchen baking a cake for her grandson's birthday. The student was impressed that in spite of her severe lumbar arthritis with a history of fractures, she was still able to enjoy the ability to create a memory for her family. Here, the student could see that with proper medication management and periodic follow-up with lab work and additional testing, a person can maintain a good and valuable quality of life. This student was excited to be put in complete charge of the house call, including taking a full history of medications and prescriptions and planning of lab work and X-rays. The experience was a great opportunity for the student's individual development.

There are certain things I teach my students to look out for during a house call visit. Since many house call patients are elderly, safety in the home becomes an important issue. Assessing fall risks is essential to the visit. It is important for the student to observe the potential danger of a fall by having a keen eye for furniture placement, noting area rugs or staircases that may present a problem. Students are asked to observe family dynamics as well as note any socioeconomic difficulties the patient may have. I'd like to note here that it is important to recognize that many housebound patients are being taken care of by family members. These selfless warriors make many sacrifices to keep their loved ones safe and in good health. Professional caregivers also perform an invaluable service. In those rare circumstances where signs of physical or mental abuse of the patient are seen, protective services for the elderly must be informed. I have the student take an active role if this should occur. Finally, after the house call, I encourage students to follow up and schedule another visit or to speak with the patient by phone.

House calls are a unique and wonderful way for student doctors to bond with their patients. They are able to get a glimpse of what life is like for them. The students' experiences can range from witnessing a person trying to "walk" across the living room using her hands on one visit to enjoying a cup of tea and homemade cookies on the next. The home visit represents a wonderful value for the student's growth and broadens his appreciation of the beauty of medicine.

CHAPTER 16

Final Evaluation

We have come to the last week of the four-week rotation. I have been carefully and perhaps secretly observing the student regarding his or her growth and maturity. I ask myself this question: Is this student a potential physician of quality, someone I'd want to care for me, my family, and other future patients? Certainly, I do not expect perfection at this point; however, if I have been able to plant the seeds of understanding regarding what I feel is required to be a physician in our complex society, the rotation has been a success. One needs only to witness the enthusiasm on the face of the student as a sick individual presents to the office. The student's true fulfillment in caring for the patient is clear. His writeups are carefully thought out, with the history of the present illness more complete, the differential diagnosis clearer, and pertinent negatives well delineated. The physicals are also more orderly and the ability to define problem lists and reasonable resolutions and plans continues to improve.

I witness the students' confidence and make sure they are humble in vocalizing that knowledge. I hope I have taught them that it's all right to forget and relearn, refresh their memories, and that they can always look things up. I ask myself: Have I been a good role model by giving them the opportunity to observe as I interact with my patients? Yet it is important that they are aware that I am by no means a perfect standard of reference: All of us have a unique approach to caring and dealing with patients. Each of us must find his own niche in the practice of medicine.

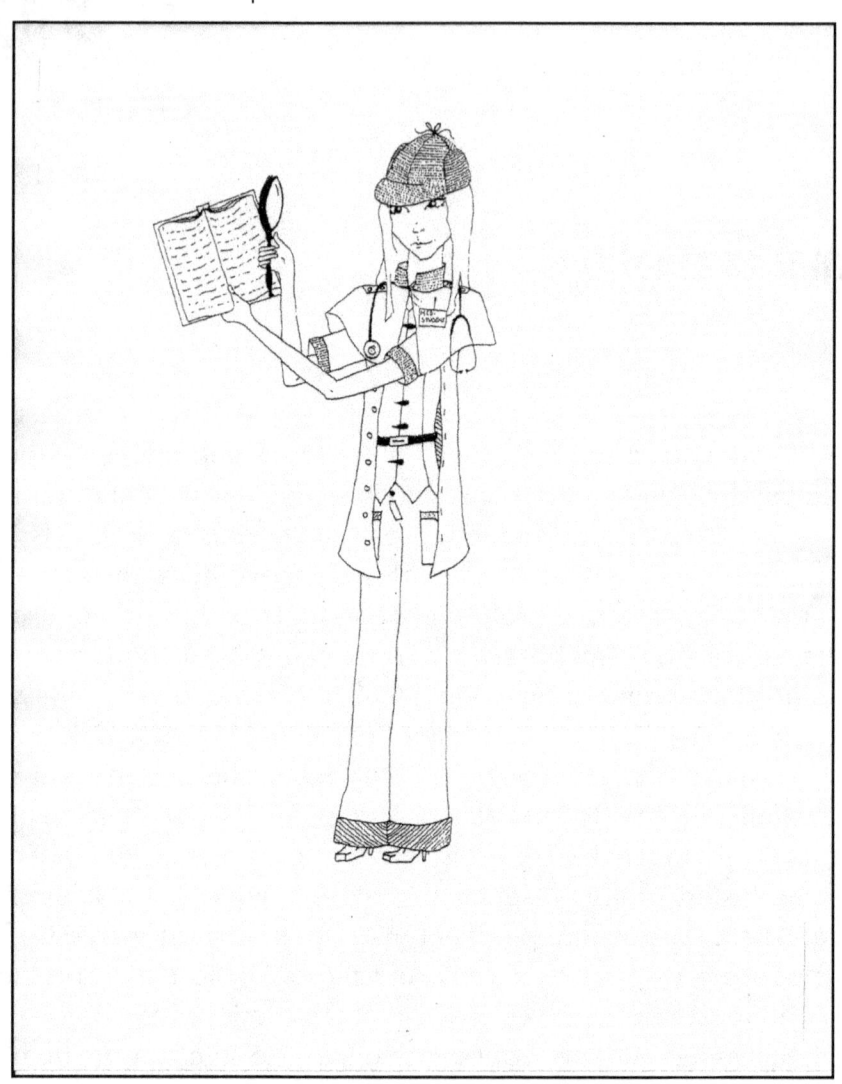

"Dr." Sherlock Holmes is on the case!

I have taught many of the finest students in the country, observing them as they move from day 1 to day 28. I see the students' professionalism grow, their demeanor evolve, as they learn to speak with patients and act in the role of physician. Conscientiousness is improved. There is more of a hunger to pinpoint the necessary data like our investigator Sherlock Holmes, and like him, they know when and how to call on their consultants. They have been drilled on lab data results and what is required in different disease processes like diabetes, hypertension, and in the patient who is complaining of fatigue. They are speaking the right language to their patients; phone calls to find out how the patient is doing (perhaps to a patient who has an unstable home situation) are almost automatic. A rapport with their patients has been developed, along with a clear sense of trust. They have the ability to teach their patients about necessary preventive screening, to discuss psychological and social issues and family problems. The students have been introduced to office procedures and have a sense of competence as they continue to improve their technique.

Most importantly, I hope that each student has learned that his sense of compassion must always be at the forefront of his work in healing patients medically and psychologically. Although, of course, there are varying degrees of growth in every student, the seeds have been planted. His fear of learning the vast amounts of medical information that are required of him has been eased. He knows that even in our sometimes difficult society, he can make a difference to his fellow man.

Figure 1

Syllabus for Primary Health-Care Rotation with Dr. Zaretzky: What to Expect ━━━━━━━━━━━━

I. Reading topics

Each student will be given a list of reading assignments that includes important topics relating to common diseases seen in clinical practice.

II. Types of visits

    A. Brief: 5–15 minutes, 1–2 problems (example: sore throat)

    B. Intermediate: 15–30 minutes, 3–4 problems (example: pneumonia)

    C. Extended: 30–45 minutes, 4–5 problems (example: abdominal or chest pain)

    D. Complete physical: 45–75 minutes (example: total examination of a 55 year old with HTN, DM, and hypercholesterolemia)

III. What is expected of students

Each student must develop a database and ask appropriate questions on history so as to develop differential diagnosis. Physical exam should be limited to those organ systems that will answer patient's chief complaint.

IV. Case discussions

Each student must come out of exam room and discuss patient with attending or medical resident. A brief presentation of the case must be given (less than 3 minutes). Students are expected to know the side effects of all medications given and to look up drug interactions. The attending will then go into room with patient and student, where again a brief history and physical will be done, after which the attending and student will discuss differential diagnosis and therapy. The student must use these discussions to build on his/her differential diagnosing abilities.

V. Laboratory data

Students are required to request lab data ordered by the team for review and rectify any abnormalities.

VI. Case presentations

Students will present and write up three cases per week: one brief, one intermediate, and one complete physical. These must be handed to Dr. Zaretzky weekly.

VII. Prescription writing

Students will be asked to write prescriptions under the direct supervision of the attending.

VIII. Patient followings

Each patient seen by students will be called at home (when possible) with lab results or as a follow-up to see how they are feeling. Better? Worse?

IX. Testing

Students will have at least two exams in a month's rotation, at two weeks and at four weeks. These will consist of theoretical cases and functional information such as causes of hyperkalemia, side effects of diuretics, etc.

X. Billing

Students should not make any notes on billing sheet.

XI. Office notes

Students should write a detailed note on each patient seen. If it is not complete at the end of the first visit due to lack of time, students must stay until note is completed.

XII. Time requirements

Hours depend on business of office. Attending may enter a room before a student has finished his/her exam. Office patient flow is an important part of training.

XIII. Procedures
Students will assist in performing the following: 1) skin biopsies, 2) flexible sigmoidoscopies, 3) excision of minor skin lesions and incision and draining of abscesses.

XIV. Questions
Please ask questions, as this shows the necessary inquisitiveness needed in medicine. Conscientiousness is a definite asset to being successful.

XV. The office visit
Don't be afraid of the patient and remember that you usually know more than they do. LISTEN to the patient rather than doing most of the talking. Most of the patients will not throw you out. If you see a sign on the door saying "no students," go to another room. Most patients will welcome you and appreciate the time you spend. Upon entering the room, say hello and introduce yourself by name and as a medical student. If the patient has no objections, proceed with history and physical exam.

XVI. Examination rules
If you are a male, never examine a female patient without another female present (i.e., breast and pelvic exams).

XVII. Interpretation of tests
Students will be learning about EKGs, X-rays, and interpretation of lab data.

XVIII. __ATTITUDE__
An eager-to-learn attitude goes a long way. What you know is important, but how hard you try is also quite important in evaluations.

XIX. Nursing homes and hospital care
Time permitting, you may go with Dr. Zaretzky to nursing homes. You will be writing notes in the chart and familiarizing yourself with the chart itself. Each student will be assigned several hospital cases. Students must see them each day and write a progress note prior to going to the office. Please be at the office between 9:30 and 10:00 a.m. Dr. Zaretzky will see hospital patients with you at some time during the day. New admissions will always be seen by the students.

Please write no more than 3 pages and try to develop your own opinions in each case.

XX. Attendance

If you have a good reason not to come in, such as an interview, please give Dr. Zaretzky advance notice.

XXI. Team approach

Remember, you are an integral part of Dr. Zaretzky's team. You will be responsible for the patient and essentially will be the "doctor" as well as the student. There will always be support for the fledgling student.

XXII. Presentation of topics

Students may be assigned topics, like multiple myeloma or COPD, and may be asked to present them to the team.

XXIII. Office attire

Have a professional look, i.e., wear a white coat and have needed equipment.

XXIV. Approach

Don't be afraid of what you don't know. We are all learning by ourselves and from each other, gathering bits of information that will build with time. Develop a humble approach to medicine. Caring and compassion for patients goes a long way.

XXV. Lunches

Bring your own lunch, or you can go out for 45 minutes. Let us know when you are leaving.

XXVI. House calls

Time permitting, students will see patients with Dr. Zaretzky for house calls.

Good luck, and hopefully your "Z" experience will be a great one. As a student, you can make a difference in your patient's well being both medically and psychologically.

Rotation Reading Topics

Weeks 3–4	Weeks 3–4
1. pneumonia	1. rheumatoid arthritis
2. headaches—causes	2. Wegener's granulomatosis
3. hypotension	3. polymyositis/ dermatomyositis
4. hypothyroidism	4. renal tumors
5. hyperthyroidism	5. paraneoplastic syndromes
6. hyponatremia	6. VIP syndromes
7. sore throats and treatments	7. MEN's
8. ear infections and treatments	8. osteoporosis
9. renal failure	9. breast cancer
10. sarcoidosis	10. Hodgkin's disease
11. leukemia	11. lymphoma
12. chest pain	12. hepatitis C
13. disorders of the esophagus	13. chronic alcoholism
14. peptic ulcer disease	14. hepatitis B
15. cardiomyopathy	15. splenomegaly—causes
16. pericarditis	16. polycythemia vera
17. right lower quadrant abdominal pain	17. secondary polycythemia
18. left lower quadrant abdominal pain	18. COPD
19. nephritis	19. asthma
20. urinary tract infections	20. hemochromatosis
21. papillary necrosis—causes	21. health screening
22. hypercalcemia	22. left upper quadrant abdominal pain

23. low back pain—causes	23. right upper quadrant abdominal pain
24. diabetes mellitus	24. Dressler's syndrome
25. hypoglycemia	25. myocardial infarctions
26. hypokalemia	26. CHF
27. hyperkalemia	27. eating disorders
28. carpal tunnel syndrome	28. depression
29. TB	29. anxiety
30. degenerative joint disease	30. sexual dysfunction
31. fever of unknown origin	31. hematuria
32. Lyme disease and tick-borne illnesses	32. renal stones
33. amyloidosis	33. pyuria and pyelonephritis
34. meningitis	34. hypercholesterolemia
35. Legionnaires' disease	35. side effects of TB drugs
36. hypertension—causes and treatment	36. drug abuse
37. HIV/AIDS	37. delirium tremens
38. side effects of diuretics and HTN meds	38. arthralgia—causes
39. chronic fatigue syndrome	39. mononucleosis and EBV
40. insulinoma	40. cerebral concussion
41. anemia—microcytic/normocytic	41. anemia—macrocytic
42. acidosis/alkalosis	

Figure 2

Question-and-Answer Test 1

1. A 59-year-old white male presents to the office for a follow-up visit. He has a known history of diabetes mellitus type 2 and hypertension. His medications include glyburide 5 mg po qd, metformin 1000 mg po bid, and simvastatin 20 mg po qd. He has a blood pressure of 160/110, pulse = 80 and regular, respiratory rate = 15, temperature = 98 °F. HEENT: no jaundice or cyanosis. Neck: no JVD, thyroid not enlarged. Lungs: clear. Heart: regular rhythm, no murmurs, S3, or S4. Pulses 2+ DP and PTs. He has a history of urticaria to beestings. Labs: BS = 240, cholesterol = 280, and LDL = 168. **What medications will you choose for the patient's hypertension, diabetes mellitus, and high cholesterol? What will you teach your patient in the exam room?**

2. A 42-year-old black female presents with left pleuritic chest pain, fever of 103 °F, and cough productive of yellow sputum. She has a known history of hypertension on amlodipine 5 mg po qhs. Her speech is slurred, and she states that her left foot is cold and she has trouble speaking. PE: pulse = 140 irregularly irregular, BP =

160/100, respiratory rate = 30. HEENT: no cyanosis. Neck: + JVD, no bruit, + thyroid enlargement; a thyroid nodule is palpable in the right lobe. Heart: irregularly irregular rate of 140, III/VI murmur is heard in the mitral area. Abdomen: liver = 16 cm, spleen palpable. Legs: 2+ edema, left foot cold. Neuro: R arm and R leg weakness IV/V, Babinski: upgoing right, downgoing left. Labs—CBC: WBC = 17,800K with 90 segs, H/H = 10/29, normocytic normochromic indices. BS = 285. BUN/Cr = 60/3. Urine: +RBC casts. Stool: guaiac positive (occult blood). **What are your thoughts? Do a workup and design a treatment plan. You are the doctor: Call your consults.**

3. A 90-year-old white female gets up from her favorite living room chair and has sudden right hip pain and falls. She sustains a right intertrochanteric hip fracture. She drinks four shots of vodka per day and has smoked two packs of cigarettes per day for 70 years. Her menopause was at 50 years old. She has a history of COPD and takes prednisone 5 mg po qd, albuterol prn, and ipatropium inhaled qid. Her last M.D. told her that she has cirrhosis of the liver. She is 5'11" tall and 105 lb. **Discuss your proposed treatments. What are some causes of osteoporosis? What will you advise her after hip surgery? What could she have done to avoid this condition 40 years ago?**

4. Your very chatty 82-year-old aunt is sitting at the Thanksgiving table. She found out that you are a medical student and says she is "blind in the left eye." **What questions do you ask her? What are the causes?**

5. List the reasons you want to be a doctor and how you want to make a difference.

6. Define:
a) Cardiomyopathy, b) BOOP syndrome, c) PIE syndrome.

7. Benign monoclonal gammopathy vs. multiple myeloma. **What is the difference?**

8. A 50-year-old obese white woman presents to your office and states, "I'm always tired." **What are your thoughts? What history will you obtain? What will be your possible workup?**

9. What are 10 causes of headache and how do you tell the difference through patient's history and diagnostic testing if required?

10. What are 10 causes of painful joints in the hands and how do you tell the difference in the clinical presentations of arthritis?

11. Give 10 causes of chest pain: **Describe the clinical scenario for each including age at onset, symptoms, and what relieves it.**

12. A 62-year-old female presents with two months of cough nonproductive of sputum. There is no weight loss, fever, chills, or hemoptysis. She has diabetes mellitus, DOE, PND, and orthopnea. You palpate a slightly hardened area in the left breast (upper outer quadrant). Her BP is 220/130, BS = 355, total cholesterol = 440, HDL = 14, LDL = 220, TG = 150. Stools are positive for occult blood. Urine has 2+ albumin and you see red blood cell casts. Chest X-ray shows bilateral hilar adenopathy. LFTs: AST = 350, ALT = 150, alk. phos. = 460, total bili. = 4. **What is your differential diagnosis and problem list?**

13. A 35-year-old black female presents with 50 lb weight loss in nine months. She has bulky, cheesy, foul-smelling stools that float on top of the water. She has low iron, low B12, and low carotene.
a) List two viruses that cause this.
b) List two enzyme deficiencies.
c) List two surgeries.
d) List two cancers.

Question-and-Answer Test 2

1. A 78-year-old white female with type 2 diabetes mellitus enters the office and blacks out in the waiting room. Her medications include metformin, glipizide, and pioglitazone HCl. Labs: BS = 460 (75–115 mg/dL), HbA1c = 9 (3.8–6.4%), BUN/Cr = 80/3 (7–18/<1.5 mg/dL). EKG: A-Fib at 130 (new). **What is your plan if the physical exam is as follows**—Vitals: BP = 70/50, P = 130 (irregularly irregular), temp = 103 °F. HEENT: pale + cyanotic + JVD + thyroid nodule. Heart: irregularly irregular, III/VI, murmur of mitral regurgitation heard in the mitral area. Abdomen: + tenderness RUQ. Extremities: no pulses DP/PT on right (cold extremity). Rectal exam: mass palpable at 6 cm, negative for blood.

2. A 32-year-old white female wedding planner with type 1 diabetes mellitus was dancing exuberantly at a recent wedding and blacked out. Meds: insulin glargine 45 U hs, regular insulin sliding scale (RISS), sumatriptan, atorvastatin 40 mg, enalapril 10 mg, ASA 81 mg. EKG: ST elevation in leads II, III, AVF. HEENT: left cervical lymphadenopathy (biopsy is suspicious for lymphoma). She wakes up with left hemiparesis and facial droop. She has a history of migraines (six/month). Additionally, she has had three previous pregnancies, all lost within 4 months. **What are your thoughts?**

3. An 87-year-old white female dances the night away at a recent Florida party with two gentlemen. She consumes eight gin-and-tonics, falls on the balcony, and fractures her hip. Meds: asthma—prednisone 10 mg qd, albuterol inhaler prn; GERD—lansoprazole prn; calcium 500 mg qd and ASA 81 mg qd. She went through menopause at age 48. She is 5'10" and thin (120 lb). CBC: H/H = 7/23, MCV = 62. Stools: + for occult blood. Thoracic spine: + compression fractures. **What could you have done to prevent the above? What do you do now? What is the workup now to clear her for surgery as a consult?**

4. What are 12 side effects of hydrochlorothiazide?

5. A 73-year-old white female presents to the office with joint stiffness. Meds: APAP, 16 ibuprofen/day, levothyroxine (for hypothyroidism). She has lost pigment in her hands and legs, has an Hct of 23, with early satiety and 25 lb weight loss over 6 months. **What are your thoughts? What is the workup?**

6. A 40-year-old black male comes in with LUQ, epigastric, and RUQ pain + vomiting bright red blood after retching 12 times. His labs reveal—CBC: WBC = 13,000 (4500–11,000), H/H = 10/25 (13.5–17.5 g/dL/41.0–53.0%). Lipase: 8050 (0–160 U/L). ABG: pH = 7.57 (7.38–7.44), PCO_2 = 25 (35–45 mmHg), PO_2 = 60 (80–100 mmHg). The physical exam shows: temp = 101 °F, P = 130 (regular), R = 30, BP = 90/70. HEENT: + jaundice, no JVD, + thyroid nodule (left lobe). Chest: left lung dull to percussion with diminished breath sounds. Heart: R = 130 (regular), no murmurs, S3 heard. **What is your plan? Thoughts?**

7. What are 10 questions to ask your 32-year-old Hispanic female patient who has a cough?

8. Give 10 reasons why your 68-year-old white female patient who lost her husband one year ago has chronic headaches, is moody, and is always tired. She takes 12 ASA/day. She has flank pain. She drinks 12 beers/day and her husband was a bisexual IV drug abuser who died of TB. She has lost 25 lb in the past 6 months.

9. What are four causes of hypokalemia and eight causes of hyperkalemia?

10. Give side effects of a) ACE inhibitors and b) statins. Causes of glomerulonephropathy? Define nephrotic syndrome.

11. What are eight causes of eosinophilia?

12. Give two causes of eosinophils in the urine.

13. List 12 causes of urticaria.

Figure 3

Matching Section

1) SIADH	A) Fasting for 72 hr tests for this, plus C-peptide
2) Opioids	B) Renal adjustment for CO2 retaining COPD patient
3) Bartter's syndrome	C) Pancreatitis
4) Doxycycline	D) Non-gap acidosis, elevated Cl
5) PTH-related protein	E) Carcinoma in situ in ulcerative colitis
6) TIAs, beta-blocker helps	F) Papillary necrosis
7) Atypical chest pain	G) Paroxysmal atrial tachycardia (PAT)
8) Elevated osteoclast activating factor	H) Fecal impaction
9) Elevated triglycerides	I) Chlorpropamide
10) RA	J) "Chitlins" (pork intestine)
11) Hodgkin's/Hep. B/PAN	K) Sarcoidosis

12) Girdle stiffness and decreased range of motion	L) Pill esophagitis
13) Change in mental status/ SIADH/elevated LFTs/GI complaints	M) Elevated renin and aldosterone, normal BP
14) Elevated glycohemoglobins (HbA1c)	N) Mitral valve prolapse
15) Insulinoma	O) TNF receptor blocker helpful
16) Eosinophilia	P) Temporal arteritis
17) Reverse pulmonary edema pattern on chest X-ray	Q) Headaches
18) Metabolic alkalosis	R) "NAACP"
19) Diabetes mellitus and renal disease	S) PIE syndrome
20) Diarrhea in the convalescent home	T) Renal cancer
21) Acetazolamide and Crohn's disease	U) Breast cancer
22) End-to-end anastomosis	V) Women may present like this
23) Lupus pernio—"panda bear sign" on gallium scan	W) Na+ of 120
24) Yersinia	X) Glomerulonephritis
25) MAI, Isospora belli	Y) Legionella
26) Urticaria (hives)	Z) 2-hr postprandial blood sugar = 180
27) Colectomy needed	A') Hypoaldo hyporenin syndrome (Type IV RTA)
28) Hyperkalemia	B') Colon polyp-stalk with cancer in situ
29) Syncope	C') HIV infection

30) Elevated TSH before pheochromocytoma	D') Hep. B/tight clothes/ exercise-induced
31) Alcoholism/sickle cell disease/NSAIDS	E') Medical residents and interns
	F') MEN syndrome (Sipple's)

*Answer key: 1 = I or W, 2 = Q, 3 = M, 4 = L, 5 = T, 6 = N, 7 = V, 8 = U, 9 = C or W, 10 = O, 11 = X, 12 = P, 13 = Y, 14 = Z, 15 = A, 16 = R, 17 = S, 18 = B, 19 = A', 20 = H, 21 = D, 22 = B', 23 = K, 24 = J, 25 = C', 26 = D', 27 = E, 28 = E', 29 = G or N, 30 = F', 31 = F.